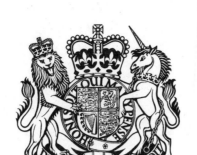

THE INTERIM RESPONSE
TO
THE REPORT OF THE
BSE INQUIRY

BY HM GOVERNMENT IN
CONSULTATION WITH THE DEVOLVED
ADMINISTRATIONS

Presented to Parliament by the Minister of Agriculture,
Fisheries and Food by Command of Her Majesty, February 2001

CM   5049

Gratis

CONTENTS

EXECUTIVE SUMMARY

The Government is issuing this Interim Response to the Report of The BSE Inquiry to provide a basis for consultations and discussions and to enable interested parties to contribute to the development of the final response. It discusses the main cross-cutting themes emerging from the Inquiry Report and provides detailed comments on the 167 individual lessons for the future.

Chapter 1, the Introduction, sets out the background to the BSE Inquiry Report and this Interim Response.

Chapter 2 summarises the current position on the BSE epidemic in the UK, and notes recent developments in Europe.

Chapter 3 explains that the care package provided for victims of vCJD and their families has been enhanced by new arrangements made in August 2000 and further improved following publication of the Report.

Chapter 4, on Science and Government, sets out the way the Government is developing its approach to obtaining scientific advice, through guidance on the operation of scientific advisory committees, and how it is seeking to improve the management of departmental research programmes. The role of the Chief Scientific Adviser and his part in departmental co-ordination and the effective use of science and research is also covered.

Chapter 5, on Openness, shows how the Food Standards Agency and its commitment to openness represents a major step forward since the period reviewed by the Inquiry. It notes how departments are becoming more open following the Freedom of Information Act 2000, and the steps being taken to embed a more positive approach to putting information in the public domain.

Chapter 6, on Risk and Uncertainty, explains the Government's position on the management and communication of risk, it explains that the Government's approach is to take action to manage risks where appropriate, in proportion to the risk and to make available to the public sufficient information so that individuals can make their own choices. It sets out progress since the late 1980s when the uncertainties of BSE were first addressed. The importance of further training is recognised, and the need for officials across government to become more familiar with handling risk.

Chapter 7, on Good Government, notes the relevance of the Inquiry's comments to the Modernising Government agenda and points particularly to the further impetus the Inquiry has given to more open, inclusive behaviour by departments and officials. Arrangements for joined-up working – between professionals and administrators, between departments and between Whitehall and the devolved administrations – continue to be strengthened and made more effective. This chapter also deals with the roles and responsibilities of the Government's key professional advisers in the areas of human and animal disease – the Chief Medical Officer and the Chief Veterinary Officer.

Chapter 8 discusses the Legislative Framework and the powers available to deal with potential hazards such as BSE.

Chapter 9 summarises the key issues for consultation, on which views from all parties would be particularly welcome.

Annex I covers each of the 167 individual lessons identified in the BSE Inquiry Report. It explains the Government's position on each of these lessons – what action has been taken, what is planned and how others will be involved in the final outcome.

CHAPTER 1 – INTRODUCTION

Introduction

1.1. BSE is a national tragedy. It has had damaging and far reaching effects. It has led to the emergence of vCJD and the deaths of more than 80 people. It has had a serious impact on tens of thousands of people whose livelihoods depend on the rearing of livestock and the processing and manufacturing of meat products.

1.2. The BSE Inquiry was established by the Government to review the emergence of BSE and variant CJD and the action taken in response to it. Its Report was published by the Government on 26 October 2000.

1.3. The Government welcome the Report, which is the result of an important and thorough Inquiry, conducted over the best part of three years. Immediate action has been taken on a number of fronts, most importantly work aimed at improving the care of vCJD victims and support for their families. In addition, the Government has now had the opportunity to consider carefully the many findings of the Report and to study the lessons that flow from them. They are important findings and they address some fundamental questions for public administration. This Response explains how the Government intends to address the key issues.

1.4. All the devolved administrations were fully involved in developing this Response, and are taking action where appropriate.

The BSE Inquiry

1.5. The BSE Inquiry was set up by the Government in December 1997:

"To establish and review the history of the emergence and identification of BSE and new variant CJD in the United Kingdom, and of the action taken in response to it up to 20 March 1996. To reach conclusions on the adequacy of that response, taking into account the state of knowledge at the time; and to report on these matters by 31 December 1998 to the Minister of Agriculture, Fisheries and Food, the Secretary of State for Health and the Secretaries of State for Scotland, Wales and Northern Ireland."

1.6. The Inquiry was led by Lord Phillips of Worth Matravers, Master of the Rolls, with Mrs June Bridgeman CB and Professor Malcolm Ferguson-Smith FRS.

1.7. The Government received the Inquiry's Report at the beginning of October 2000 and published it on 26 October 2000. The Rt. Hon Nick Brown MP, Minister of Agriculture, Fisheries and Food, made a statement in the House of Commons (Annex VI), on behalf of the Government, thanking the Committee for their work and welcoming the findings of the Report.

Developments since 1996

1.8. The Inquiry looked at the period up to 20 March 1996. Since that time the Government has introduced some very significant changes which impact on agriculture and food safety and on the protection of the consumer. The most important are:

- the creation of the Food Standards Agency (FSA) as an independent, non-Ministerial department responsible for food safety policy in the United Kingdom. The Agency has as its central aim the protection of public health;

- the establishment of the devolved legislatures and administrations;

- the "Modernising Government" and Civil Service Reform agendas;

- steps taken by the Office of Science and Technology to improve the Government's use of science and expert committees, such as issuing the "Guidelines 2000" and a proposed code of practice.

Details of these and other relevant Government policies are available via a range of publications and Government web-sites; a selection is included at Annex IV.

Action following the Inquiry Report

1.9.   On receiving the Inquiry Report, the Government took immediate steps to improve the care of vCJD patients, and to begin working on a compensation scheme for victims and their families. The enhanced care arrangements are set out in Chapter 3. Discussions with the families of vCJD victims about a compensation scheme are underway and interim payments will be made.

1.10.   The Government has also acted on the Inquiry's conclusions about the origin of BSE. The Minister of Agriculture, Fisheries and Food has announced that Professor Gabriel Horn will chair an independent review of the current scientific understanding, including emerging findings, of the origin of the BSE epidemic. Findings from the review will be considered by the Spongiform Encephalopathy Advisory Committee (SEAC), and published. They will contribute to the Government's final response to the Inquiry Report.

1.11.   The review of the criticisms of serving civil servants led by Sheila Forbes, a Civil Service Commissioner, has now been completed. Sheila Forbes has recommended to the Permanent Secretaries of the departments involved that there is no justification for disciplinary action to be taken against any serving civil servant. They have accepted this recommendation and the civil servants involved have been informed.

The Government's Interim Response

1.12.   This Response focuses on the key themes that come out of the Inquiry Report. Although the Report looks primarily at how the Government of the day responded to the challenge of BSE and vCJD, it raises much wider issues that affect the whole process of Government, across all departments. There are a number of major cross-cutting topics which run right through the Report: the way in which the Government uses scientific advisory committees and expert advice; openness; the importance of a consistent and proportionate approach to risk management; and the conduct of government, focusing on the importance of good co-ordination and a rigorous approach to policy development and implementation.

1.13. The chapters dealing with these themes are forward looking, but they also take the opportunity to explain developments since 1996. They show how the Government is already using the Report's findings as a way of giving more priority to the Modernising Government agenda, the work of the Office of Science and Technology on the best use of science in government and the development of a Government Statement on Risk. This Response recognises the need for government departments to change the way they operate, with the emphasis on securing positive changes in behaviour rather than in policy, structure or machinery.

1.14. Detailed responses to the 167 lessons in the Inquiry Report are set out in Annex I. There is information about the Government's position on each of the lessons, what action has already been taken, what is planned and how others will be involved in the final outcome.

Consultation

1.15. The key developments since March 1996 are reflected in this Response. Proposals for further action indicate the direction in which the Government plans to go to implement the Inquiry Report. But this is an interim response and is intended as a basis for consultation and discussion so that all interested parties can contribute to the development of the final response. In parallel the devolved administrations are also considering the Report in the context of their own responsibilities.

1.16. Information on how to register comments on the Government's Interim Response is set out at Annex VII.

1.17. The Government will also be seeking views and comments on the issues raised by the Inquiry's Report through a programme of meetings and discussions with interested parties.

CHAPTER 2 – THE BSE EPIDEMIC – A SUMMARY

2.1.   The BSE epidemic in the UK reached its peak early in 1993. Since then the number of cases has decreased very significantly. There are now around 30 new BSE suspect cases being reported each week – at the peak of the epidemic there were over 1,000. Extensive facts and figures on BSE since 20 March 1996 can be found in the six-monthly Progress Reports published by MAFF (the December 2000 edition will be published shortly), and there is a range of material accessible via the MAFF and FSA websites.

2.2.   The stringent controls now in place in the United Kingdom have been built up over a number of years. A summary of present controls is provided at Annex II. The Food Standards Agency undertook a review of BSE controls in relation to the food chain and published their report on 20 December 2000. The main conclusion was that none of the three major BSE controls should be relaxed; these controls are the Animal Feed Ban, removal of Specified Risk Material (SRM) and the Over Thirty Months Scheme. The Government acknowledges this and remains fully committed to maintaining all the controls needed to protect human and animal health and to eliminate BSE.

2.3.   Epidemiologists at Oxford University have recently estimated that less than one BSE infected bovine within 12 months of developing clinical disease will have entered the human food chain in Great Britain in the year 2000. This is the result of controls such as the 1988 ruminant feed ban and the 1996 ban on feeding mammalian meat and bone meal to all farmed animals (which have led to the decline in the BSE epidemic) and the operation of the over 30 month rule (which restricts cattle from entry into the food chain). By comparison, more than two million cattle are slaughtered for food annually. The remaining risk from animals entering the food chain is very small. Nonetheless, parts of cattle which are most likely to carry BSE infectivity are removed at the slaughterhouse and may not be used for human consumption.

2.4.   Following a rise in the incidence of BSE in other parts of Europe, the Community has recently stepped up precautionary measures across the EU. These substantially follow UK experience and controls. They include strengthened SRM and feed controls, and a prohibition on the sale for human consumption of cattle aged over 30 months unless the carcass has been tested negatively for BSE.

CHAPTER 3 – CARE FOR vCJD VICTIMS

3.1.　This Chapter reports progress on taking forward the Government's decision, announced in the Minister of Agriculture's statement on 26 October (Annex VI), to improve the care available to people who are suffering from vCJD, and to provide a compensation scheme for victims and their families.

Findings of the Inquiry

3.2.　The Inquiry noted that standards of care and support for families varied widely and suggested that improvements were needed, including:

- as speedy as possible a diagnosis of vCJD;

- informed and sympathetic advice to relatives about the future course of the disease and the needs of the patient;

- speedy assistance for those who wished to care for the victim at home (needs often include aids for the care of the disabled, modification to the home, financial assistance and respite care);

- a co-ordinated care package which addresses the needs of the victims and their families; and, if requested

- a suitable institutional environment for a young person, incapacitated and terminally ill.

Problems with the Care of vCJD Victims

3.3.　People with vCJD deteriorate rapidly. Degenerative diseases of the young are rare and the structure of the health service makes no special provision for them. Problems have arisen because families have not been enabled to care for vCJD victims at home or because inadequate care packages have been provided.

Government Action

3.4.　In August 2000 the Department of Health issued guidance to the NHS and Social Services departments making it clear that care for people suffering from vCJD should be well organised with a proper care package put into place as soon as possible. This package should include the appointment of a key worker for each patient to oversee the development of their care plan. The guidance stressed the need for the key worker to liaise with the care co-ordinator at the CJD Surveillance Unit who provides specialist expertise in CJD and acts as an information resource for carers and professionals. Similar arrangements apply in Scotland and Wales.

3.5.　Since publication of the Inquiry Report, the Department of Health has been in close contact with the Royal College of Psychiatrists, looking at ways of shortening the time taken to obtain a diagnosis of CJD. The Government has established a new national fund of £1 million to provide better care for patients suffering from all forms of CJD. This money is not intended for routine care and treatment, but will help to solve problems and overcome local difficulties over the timeliness or availability of particular services. The care package fund is already benefiting people with CJD. Two families have, or are about to receive, services supported by the fund. The care package fund is administered by the care co-ordinator at the CJD Surveillance Unit who works closely with the patient's key worker and is supported in operating the fund by additional staff employed by the CJD Surveillance Unit. The Department of Health has been working with families of CJD patients, including the Human BSE Foundation, to make sure that proposals for setting up the care package fund and the advice network described in 3.6 meet their needs.

3.6.   The Government is also establishing a "virtual" network, comprising people with direct experience of caring for sufferers of CJD. This will help to provide a ready source of information and advice for health and social care staff. Nearly all families wish to care for vCJD victims at home – the care fund will help to make this possible. Where home care is not possible, however, the key worker can make arrangements for CJD victims in a suitable hospice or neurological nursing home.

3.7.   Discussions with families of vCJD victims on a compensation scheme are underway and interim payments will be made.

The Future

3.8.   If vCJD cases increase markedly in the future, the Government will look again at how the care fund can best be operated and whether future care arrangements should operate on a regional, rather than a national basis.

CHAPTER 4 – SCIENCE AND GOVERNMENT

Introduction

4.1. This chapter is concerned with the way the Government obtains scientific advice, and how it is used in taking policy decisions. It covers the role and operation of scientific advisory committees and looks at how the Government and individual departments manage and co-ordinate their research programmes.

4.2. This represents an agenda for the UK in so far as policy and management of some aspects of science are reserved to the UK Government. Policy and management for many other aspects of science have been devolved to the administrations in Scotland, Wales and Northern Ireland. This document has been prepared as a joint exercise and the devolved administrations agree the broad thrust of this chapter, but may, in due course, adopt policy or delivery mechanisms that are different. The UK Government and the devolved administrations are committed to working together. **The Government and the devolved administrations would be interested in views on whether the answers to the questions posed in this chapter are different in relation to Scotland, Wales or Northern Ireland.**

4.3. The current organisation, which provides the structure for the development of strategic science policy, and information on the role of the Chief Scientific Adviser (CSA) are set out in Annex III.

A. Obtaining and using Scientific Advice

Findings of the Inquiry

4.4. The Inquiry's findings about obtaining and using scientific advice fall into two broad areas:

(i) The relationship between government and its advisers, with a particular focus on advisory committees. The Inquiry focuses on the need for departments to ensure that appropriate members are appointed to committees, to identify clearly and precisely their role and the scope of their advice, particularly in relation to the formulation of policy options, and to ensure that formal advice is properly and fully understood by departments.

(ii) The operation of the advisory committees themselves. Here the Inquiry focuses on the need for committees to follow formal risk assessment structures when analysing risk, to provide clear advice which identifies uncertainties, to explain their use of available information and their reasoning and to present their advice to the public in language that can be understood by the layman. The Inquiry also calls for committee members to declare potential conflicts of interest.

Present Position

4.5. The White Paper on Science, "Excellence and Opportunity", published in July 2000, sets out the Government's commitment to an independent and transparent advisory framework for science. Its launch was accompanied by:

- the publication of the "Guidelines 2000" on Scientific Advice and Policy Making. This is an updated version of the Chief Scientific Adviser's guidance, first issued in 1997, on the use by departments of scientific advice in policy making. The key messages in Guidelines 2000 make clear that departments should:

– think ahead, identifying the issues where scientific advice is needed at an early stage;

– get a ~~wide range of advice from~~ the best sources, particularly where there is scientific uncertainty; and

– publish the scientific advice they receive and all the relevant papers.

• the launch of a consultation exercise on a new Code of Practice for scientific advisory committees. The first round of consultation, aimed at identifying issues to be covered in the Code, closed in December 2000. It covered:

– transparency, including the information a committee should publish, handling of confidential information, reporting of uncertainty in advice to departments, communication to stakeholders and how to approach public consultation and dialogue;

– responsibilities of the chair, including training needs;

– responsibilities and duties of individual members, including an understanding of the committee's and their own personal role, achieving the right balance amongst representatives, changes of membership and actual or potential conflicts of interest;

– duties of the secretariat and other government officials involved with the committee;

– committee working practices, the use of research, early identification of issues, risk assessment, procedures for arriving at conclusions, exchange of information with other committees.

4.6. The Government considers that "Guidelines 2000" and the proposed new Code of Practice, which is being carefully assessed against the Inquiry's findings, provide a sound framework for addressing many of the concerns identified by the Inquiry.

4.7. "Guidelines 2000" sets out for departments how best to handle scientific advice. It provides broad principles of general application, rather than detailed rules. In the light of the Inquiry's findings, the Government believes there is scope for preparing more detailed guidance to departments on the need for them to:

• identify all the people in government with a policy interest and ensure they receive relevant information;

• take decisions as speedily as possible, but recognise when to obtain scientific advice first;

• involve relevant scientific advisory committees in contingency planning;

- retain appropriate internal scientific expertise to be able to understand scientific advice.

4.8. The Government is currently considering responses to the first round of consultation on the proposed Code of Practice for Scientific Advisory Committees. The second round of consultation, which will set out for public comment a draft text of the new Code, is expected to begin in March 2001. The final version of the Code will be published later this year. Lessons flowing from the BSE Inquiry will be an important element in the ongoing development of the Code.

4.9. The Chief Scientific Adviser (CSA) reports regularly on the implementation of the Guidelines and will continue to do so. Arrangements will also be considered for reporting on the implementation by departments of the Code of Practice. Proposals will be included in the second round for consultation.

Future Proposals

4.10. The Government proposes to invite the Chief Scientific Adviser to adopt the practice of writing to Permanent Secretaries, setting out good practice on arrangements for handling scientific advice and for managing research within their departments. These letters would be made public, providing quality standards against which departments could develop their own framework and providing the wider public with the means to judge how well their systems measured up to the latest benchmarks. The CSA's letters might also cover: ways of identifying emerging issues; co-ordination and communication within government; and evaluation and review of research proposals.

4.11. **The Government welcomes views on what else might be done to ensure that departments maintain an effective scientific advisory system.**

Departmental Scientific Expertise
Findings of the Inquiry

4.12. The Inquiry found that government should retain "in-house" sufficient expertise to ensure that departments are able to identify where there is a need for advice, frame appropriate questions, understand and critically review the advice given, and act upon it in a sensible and proportionate manner.

Current position and further proposals

4.13. The Nicholson Report on Science and Technology Activity across Government (July 1999) recommended that departments should consider collectively their needs for staff with scientific and technical backgrounds. The OST, in response to this Report, is conducting scoping and exploratory work to identify present and future needs for scientific staff and, in particular, the expertise needed to handle effectively advice from scientific advisory committees. A progress report is due to be considered by the Ministerial Science Group in Spring 2001, with a view to consultation in the summer.

Other Sources of Scientific Advice

4.14. Many of the issues raised by science go beyond national boundaries. Decisions are often made by supra-national regulatory bodies; for example, the institutions of the

European Union, informed by scientific advice commissioned, collated and analysed by groups of scientists from many countries. The EU Scientific Steering Committee is an increasingly important player in the Community's legislative work on TSEs. The Government is working to ensure that the principles underlying good scientific decision making are adopted by international bodies.

4.15. One aspect of the BSE story to which the Inquiry drew particular attention was the position of scientists who were not members of advisory committees and who had views outside the scientific mainstream. Some scientists felt that their views had not received a fair hearing.

Lacey

4.16. Publication of scientific advisory committee papers and minutes, and a greater emphasis on public consultation as issues are considered, should provide a formal opportunity for a wider range of scientists to put forward their views, and ensure more open scientific debate. This will allow those with different approaches and alternative theories to be heard before advice to Ministers is formulated and policy developed. Open calls for research proposals will also help to broaden the range of possible research projects coming forward; peer review will ensure that a high standard of research is maintained.

4.17. **The Government wants to continue to develop arrangements to ensure that a full range of scientific opinions can be heard by those developing policy and would be interested in views on how this might best be undertaken.**

What about knowledge that is not 'Scientific' in any conventional way?

B.   Managing research programmes

Findings of the Inquiry

4.18. Against the background of the very large number of research projects undertaken in response to BSE, the Inquiry noted lessons in relation to:

- the importance of effective co-ordination across departments, where there are major research programmes involving human and animal health. This might involve the appointment of a research "supremo" or committee;

- the use of an open contract tendering procedure to enhance the quality and range of proposals received;

- the need to have available contingency research funds to meet unforeseen research needs;

- the need to ensure close collaboration and joint working between organisations, and to make the best use of limited specialist expertise;

- the need to consider the extent to which research should be reviewed while in progress and whether it should be peer reviewed.

The current position and future proposals

4.19. The Government agrees there is a need for departments to review and evaluate the way they manage their research programmes and to take stock of arrangements for co-ordination. Departments are changing the way they manage research. For example MAFF has:

- for the first time put its Research Strategy for 2000-2005 out for public consultation;

- established a Science Committee which includes external stakeholders;

- strengthened its arrangements for external peer review of its research programmes; and

- is developing approaches to evaluating the impact of its research programmes.

The Government believes that changes of this sort will help to improve the quality of the research that underpins and informs key policy decisions.

4.20. In recent years, Government departments have recognised that open calls for research proposals can significantly improve the quality of their research programmes. MAFF is placing an increasing proportion of its research contracts in this way and research into TSEs was the subject of an open call for proposals in April 2000. The FSA puts its research out to competitive tender and has a well established system for reviewing R&D programmes. Although open calls for research bring benefits, departments also need to ensure that they can, in an emergency, rapidly establish research projects with a credible source; and maintain access to core capabilities.

4.21. **The Government would welcome views on the arrangements for research management and whether there are different approaches that might be tested to ensure that the high quality research necessary to inform and evaluate government policy can be procured.**

Research Strategies

4.22. The White Paper "Excellence and Opportunity" placed a commitment on departments to publish science and innovation strategies. The Ministerial Science Group will keep these strategies under review, focusing on connections and the need for good communication between departments. The Group will draw on advice from members of the Council for Science and Technology. The strategies will provide an overall framework within which research programmes can be managed and prioritised, reflecting departmental objectives and priorities.

4.23. Publication of the strategies will improve the information available to the public about the Government's research priorities and the ways in which research is managed. This will enable informed observers to understand the range of the programmes, providing an opportunity to identify any gaps in research and to suggest where additional work might usefully be carried out.

Public Availability of Research Results

4.24. The Government also plans to use increased openness to help identify areas of potential weakness in the research map at the detailed level. "Guidelines 2000" and its predecessor, the Guidelines on the Use of Scientific Advice in Policy Making, make clear that publishing the data which underpins policy decisions is both necessary and important. As a result, departments are improving their arrangements for publishing research programmes. Departments, including MAFF and the FSA, now make available reports of research and provide lists of reports on their websites, enabling people to see the scientific evidence on which policies are based.

4.25.   **The Government would welcome views on whether the proposed arrangements for the development and publication of research strategies are likely to help external observers in identifying gaps and recognising priorities in departmental research programmes.**

4.26.   The Government is also exploring how improved openness could be taken a step further, by looking at establishing a centrally run website, open to the public, providing access to information about publicly-funded R&D programmes and projects. **The Government would welcome views on whether a website of this nature should be available and, if so, what the priorities should be as to its contents.**

Delays – funding and other resources

4.27.   One thread which runs right through the Inquiry Report concerns the problems caused by delays, including areas where research projects could have been started earlier. The Inquiry argues for the need to maintain contingency funds so that departments have available a sum of money to tackle unforeseen research needs.

4.28.   The Government agrees with the need to move fast to tackle newly identified risks. Some departments have contingency funds under the control of Chief Scientists – along the lines that the Inquiry suggests. These can be pressed into use very rapidly. For example, to meet the urgent need for more research on prostate cancer the Department of Health will spend an extra £1 million from its existing R&D budget in 2000/2001. MAFF is enlarging its TB research programme by increasing its funding from £1.7 million in 1997/98 to £5.9 million in 2001/2, drawing significantly on the Chief Scientist's budget. Other departments have different arrangements, ensuring the flexibility to switch funds to meet urgent needs for research. All departments believe that existing arrangements are sufficient once a risk has been identified and its priority for funding agreed, but consideration will be given as to any further action needed.

4.29.   The ability to set up research projects quickly also depends on the availability of researchers with the right expertise and access to the right facilities. Animal disease research requires very specialised facilities. The existence of a strong science base is vital in ensuring that such resources are available when needed, as is access to the key facilities and expertise which are provided through the public sector research establishments.

Horizon Scanning

4.30.   The major issue in ensuring that research can be initiated in good time is the early identification of any possible emerging risk, including ways of reaching agreement on its relative importance and on the need for early action to address it. Horizon scanning, such as that undertaken by the National Horizon Scanning Centre (NHSC) for the Department of Health in relation to new and emerging health technologies, is one example of how departments are seeking to ensure they are able to understand new research needs and to establish agreement on how best to address them. Where issues cross departmental responsibilities, the CSA and OST have a role in facilitating co-ordination.

4.31. **The Government already undertakes "horizon scanning" for possible new risks. What other approaches to identifying potential risks would be useful?**

Co-ordination of Research Programmes

4.32. There is now a significant degree of co-ordination across departments and Research Councils in relation to the TSE research programme and in other fields.

4.33. Co-ordination of TSE research is achieved through the TSE Joint Funders Co-ordination Group and the High Level Committee for TSE Research. The Funders Group aims to ensure a coherent research strategy, addressing high priority issues of national importance. Its website[1] lists all publicly funded TSE research in the UK. The Group sponsors meetings and conferences to monitor progress and organises joint calls for proposals in key research areas. The High Level Committee maintains an overview of progress, ensuring that mechanisms are in place to implement the agreed strategy and that barriers to progress can be identified and overcome. The Committee provides regular reports on progress to the Prime Minister.

4.34. The CSA is responsible for ensuring the overall quality of scientific advice to Government, with a role in overseeing the proper co-ordination of research programmes between departments and the Research Councils. The Government recognises the need to keep these arrangements under review. The last major review was published in 1996 (Review of the Inter-Relationships between the Science, Engineering and Technology Expenditure of Government Departments), and the Government now plans to look at it again, and to see how its recommendations have been implemented. It is anticipated that this new review will, as a first step, look at the arrangements for the co-ordination and management of research into BSE/vCJD and other zoonoses.

4.35. Where necessary, the CSA has a responsibility to bring together departments for the purpose of research co-ordination, either through *ad hoc* or standing arrangements. A recent example is the establishment of the High Level Group on Health Genomics. This is similar to the "research supremo" function suggested by the Inquiry.

4.36. **The Government is strengthening its research arrangements as indicated above. Are there any other approaches to this that it could adopt?**

---

[1] Owned by the MRC at www.mrc.ac.uk.

CHAPTER 5 – OPENNESS

Introduction

5.1.   This chapter describes what the Government is doing to generate greater public trust in its handling of food safety and related issues. It explains the steps the Government is taking to encourage greater openness.

Findings of the Inquiry

5.2.   The Inquiry Report contains a number of key findings in relation to trust and openness:

- To establish credibility it is necessary to generate trust.

- Trust can only be generated by openness.

- Openness requires recognition of uncertainty, where it exists.

5.3.   These conclusions are strongly endorsed by the Government. The Government recognises that there has been a significant loss of public confidence in the arrangements for handling food safety and standards, due in large part to the events surrounding BSE. It is committed to a policy of open and transparent working. The aim is to provide consumers and others with timely, accurate and scientifically based information and advice, enabling people to make informed decisions and choices. The Government recognises that its efforts to build and sustain trust through openness cannot succeed unless it is fully prepared to acknowledge uncertainty in its assessments of risk.

What the Government is doing

5.4.   The Government has introduced a range of measures to achieve these objectives. It set up the Food Standards Agency (FSA) on 1 April 2000 as a major step towards improving food safety and restoring lasting confidence. The Agency operates on a UK-wide basis, responsible to all four UK administrations. Other departments have also strengthened their arrangements for communicating with the public, and are improving the quality of information they publish on risk. New freedom of information legislation, applicable to UK public bodies in England, Wales and Northern Ireland, and separate Scottish freedom of information legislation which will apply to Scottish public bodies, provides a statutory framework for greater openness across government. This makes disclosure of information the norm in all but the most exceptional cases where publication would not be in the public interest. The following paragraphs describe in more detail what is being done.

Food Standards Agency

5.5.   The Food Standards Act 1999, under which the FSA was established, explicitly addresses the issue of openness. It gives the FSA the statutory function of providing advice and information to the general public on food safety and on other interests of consumers in relation to food. It also gives the FSA wide-ranging statutory powers of disclosure in support of its advisory functions. The Act places a duty on the FSA to make public the information on which its decisions are based, so that people can reach an informed view for themselves. The Agency is required to consult, wherever possible, before acting and to promote effective links with other departments and bodies.

5.6. The Act provides an unprecedented framework for achieving greater openness in relation to food safety. Laying down basic requirements on openness, it also places a duty on the FSA to develop more detailed policies on how it will put these into practice.

5.7. The FSA has committed itself to improving measurably public confidence in the national food safety and standards arrangements. It aims to achieve this by putting the consumer first, by being open and accessible and by being an independent voice. It has published a range of detailed targets for meeting these objectives.

5.8. In addition, the FSA has published a Statement of General Objectives and Practices, showing what is being done to make its working practices open and accessible. Besides those actions that are already required under the 1999 Act, the Agency is committed to reporting annually on its openness policies and to publishing a Code of Practice on Openness setting out how it intends to implement them (a draft has been the subject of consultation).

5.9. The Code of Practice makes clear that, in relation to the Agency's powers of publication, disclosure of advice and information will be the norm. There are limited exceptions to this, including when disclosure would be unlawful. In addition, the FSA will not normally disclose information where it considers that, on balance, it would not be in the public interest. As a public authority for the purposes of the Freedom of Information Act 2000, the FSA will also be under a statutory duty to disclose information, as provided by that Act.

5.10. Besides using its powers of disclosure, the FSA has taken a number of other steps towards greater openness. These include:

- holding its Board meetings in public;

- holding open meetings with stakeholders to take views on needs and priorities;

- encouraging the use of stakeholder groups in the development of policy (e.g. in the BSE controls review);

- promoting more effective links with consumers (e.g. through the establishment of a specialist consumer liaison unit);

- consulting wherever possible before acting, using the most productive means available (the FSA has published draft guidance to its officials on how to achieve the most out of consultation so that its decisions are as well informed as possible);

- exposing research findings to peer review as the norm;

- encouraging research contractors to publish their findings;

- encouraging its advisory committees to be open at all stages of the risk assessment process and in considering risk management options;

- encouraging these committees to be as open as possible where there are commercial confidentiality constraints;

- including consumer and/or lay representatives in the membership of all its advisory committees;

- ensuring that advisory committees hold open meetings and publishing agendas, papers and minutes on the Agency's website;

- publishing brand names, where relevant, in the findings of sampling and surveillance work;

- publishing information on the activities and performance of local authority enforcers.

5.11.   The FSA aims to ensure that consumers have access to practical information and advice to enable them to make informed choices for themselves and their families.

5.12.   **The Government is interested to know whether these initiatives and the new standards for openness set by the FSA meet the challenges of public confidence in food safety and the specific lessons of BSE. Is there more that the FSA might need to do?**

Initiatives by other departments

5.13.   The Government believes in trusting the public and agrees with the Inquiry that this is both important and necessary. Other departments are following the FSA's lead in seeking greater openness and promoting dialogue, particularly when there is a degree of uncertainty. This is a central theme of the Modernising Government agenda and is reflected in the way departments are increasing stakeholder and public involvement in decisions on risk issues.

5.14.   An example of a recent initiative to strengthen public awareness of risk is the publication by the UK Health departments of a leaflet on mobile phones and health. This openly acknowledged some of the scientific uncertainties about risks to health from exposure to radio waves. The leaflet also shared with the public the rationale for adopting a "precautionary approach" in this case. MAFF is also being more open with industry when developing policy. For example, it is sharing information on animal diseases so that farmers are in a better position to manage the commercial consequences of disease outbreaks.

5.15.   There are initiatives in other areas too; several advisory committees, even those advising on purely technical matters, now have lay members. These people play a crucial role, ensuring that the science is put across in an understandable way, and scrutinising the process of enquiry to ensure that issues are clearly defined. For example, the key advisory committee on BSE and vCJD, the Spongiform Encephalopathy Advisory Committee (SEAC), has a director of the Consumers' Association as lay member.

5.16. Approaches in other areas include:

- the creation of the Agriculture and Environment Biotechnology Commission;

- the Human Genetics Commission (which has been investigating various mechanisms of communication, including open meetings and consultation via the Internet);

- the Department of Transport, Environment and the Regions' Chemical Stakeholders' Forum and Sustainable Development Commission.

5.17. The Government is also undertaking research, via the Health and Safety Executive and Department of Health, which looks at other ways of involving the public. This includes the use of consensus conferences, citizens' juries, and public opinion surveys. The results of this research will enable policy-makers to measure the effectiveness of public participation exercises against a common benchmark, so that they can assess their relative merits.

5.18. **How might departments best implement the Government's commitment to trusting the public and continue to develop ways of being open and consulting widely while developing policy?**

The Freedom of Information Act 2000

5.19. The Freedom of Information Act 2000, which received Royal Assent last November, represents a major step towards greater openness and transparency in public life. The Act creates a statutory right of access to all information held by public bodies in England, Wales and Northern Ireland, including Government departments, unless it is covered by certain, tightly defined conditions; for example, where disclosure would breach a legal duty or would not be in the public interest. Further information is available on the Home Office website.

5.20. The Information Commissioner, created by the Act, can order a public authority to disclose information, subject to a right of appeal to a Tribunal. Under the Act, departments will be required to publish and operate a publication scheme agreed with the Commissioner. The Act also provides for the Government to remove or relax laws that prevent the disclosure of certain types of information, where such rules cannot be justified. The Home Office, together with relevant departments, is currently reviewing existing bars to disclosure and will bring forward draft legislation based on the outcome of the review in due course. Section 118 of the Medicines Act 1968 and Section 28 of the Health and Safety at Work Act fall within the scope of this review.

5.21. The Scottish Executive is committed to introducing freedom of information legislation for Scottish public bodies. A consultation document has been published and a Bill is expected to be introduced to the Scottish Parliament this year, following consultation on a draft bill.

5.22. **The Government is interested in views on the effectiveness of the steps it is taking to be more open and so generate greater public trust in its handling of food safety issues. In particular:**

- **does the programme of action described in this chapter meet the need for greater openness identified by the Inquiry?**

- **should Government departments do more to secure public trust through greater openness on food safety and related issues, and if so, what in particular should they be doing?**

CHAPTER 6 – RISK AND UNCERTAINTY

Introduction

6.1. This chapter sets out the action being taken to improve assessment and management of risk. It describes proposals for revising or reinforcing existing practices dealing with risk and uncertainty in public policy-making. The term "risk" as used in this chapter is in the context of the Inquiry Report and focuses primarily on risks to public health. Risk communication is also covered in the previous chapter on Openness.

6.2. This chapter represents an agenda for the UK as a whole. Risk and uncertainty impact upon the policy and management of powers devolved to the administrations in Scotland, Wales and Northern Ireland, and this document has been prepared as a joint exercise. The devolved administrations agree the broad thrust of the chapter, but may in due course adopt policy or delivery mechanisms that are different. The UK Government and the devolved administrations are committed to working together.

Findings of the Inquiry

6.3. A number of issues were raised by the Inquiry about the handling of risk and uncertainty across government. These include:

- the application of a precautionary approach;

- the communication of risk to the public;

- the handling of risk issues where there is uncertainty;

- the enforcement of measures designed to protect public health;

- clarity about responsibility and accountability for risk management decisions; and

- interdepartmental working on risk issues.

General framework for government policies

6.4. The Government is committed to improving the way it manages risk and uncertainty. This includes making the whole risk management process more open and transparent and involving the public more fully, and improving communication to ensure that the issue of uncertainty and relative risk and how they are handled can be clearly understood by all. Effective communication needs to be an integral part of the whole process of risk analysis, including risk assessment and management. Good risk communication is a two way process, starting with consultation and continuing throughout the risk analysis.

6.5. The Government's general approach to risk is to take action where appropriate, in proportion to the risk and to make available to the public sufficient information about a risk, in a form that is easily understood, so that individuals can make their own choices. Where for example, the risks are taken involuntarily, affect

21

particularly vulnerable groups, such as children, or where the hazard is widespread, the public expects government to ensure that measures are in place to protect them. The Government recognises that only rarely can risk be eradicated and that weighing risks and benefits should be an important part of every decision.

6.6.   Government also needs to deal with issues where people perceive possible risks to health, but where the scientific evidence of harm is inconclusive. A balance needs to be struck between intervening too much, forgoing benefits and stifling people's freedom of action, and failing to help protect them sufficiently from actual or potential hazards. However this balance is struck, the aim must always be to make the reasons for risk management decisions clear to Parliament and the public.

Recent Initiatives

6.7.   The establishment of the Food Standards Agency in April 2000 and the Freedom of Information Act, passed in November 2000, are major developments in the way the Government manages and communicates risk. The FSA now has the explicit responsibility for advice and policy on the management of food safety risks. It is required by statute to protect the interests of the public as its primary aim, but also to take account of the costs and benefits of its decisions.

Government statements on Risk

6.8.   The Modernising Government Action Plan[2] committed the Government to producing a public declaration on its approach to managing risk, to be published later this year. The Government's commitment to making public how decisions about risk are reached is also reflected in the Action Plan. All departments have prepared a risk management framework. Some have already been published: the Department of Health's framework for England was published in the 1999 Public Health White Paper *Saving Lives: Our Healthier Nation* and describes some guiding principles and key steps in its approach to risk; MAFF's *Procedures for Risk Analysis* was put out for consultation with stakeholders in September 2000; the FSA has published for consultation a draft statement on its approach to risk. The Action Plan and risk frameworks will provide the public with information on how decisions about risk are made.

Training

6.9.   Departments are taking steps to improve skill levels in relation to managing and communicating risk by developing guidance and training for policy makers. Research is being commissioned to improve the Government's understanding of public perceptions and reactions to risk issues, and findings will be used to update guidance and training programmes and also in the development of policies.

6.10.   Departments are developing better training for policy makers both at the Government's Centre for Management and Policy Studies and internally. The Department of Health has introduced training on issues such as the precautionary approach, the scientific advisory process, public perception and understanding of risk issues and the role of the media. This training has commitment from senior

---

[2] Details are available on the Cabinet Office website.

management and personal input from the CMO. MAFF has set up a programme of training workshops for managers and plans a workshop for stakeholders. It has established a Risk Forum for risk practitioners across MAFF to discuss risk management issues and promote best practice.

Research

6.11. Government departments are commissioning research to ensure a better understanding of public perceptions and reactions to risk issues. And they are investigating ways of achieving greater public involvement in the risk analysis process. Examples include research on:

- The social amplification of risk (i.e. some risks scare people while larger ones do not);

- Public participation methods (e.g. focus groups, consensus conferences, citizens' juries); and

- Risk literacy and ways of improving public understanding of health risks.

Handling scientific uncertainty

6.12. The Inquiry acknowledged that in the case of BSE, where the risks to humans were not quantifiable, there was significant scientific uncertainty. Precautionary measures were applied, but there were shortcomings in implementing and monitoring the controls. The public received "mixed messages" because reassurances about the remoteness of any risk to human health tended to be accompanied by the announcement of additional measures aimed at reducing the risk still further. Since the need for these precautionary measures was not always made clear to the public, nor to those responsible for carrying them out, their potential importance to public health was devalued. The Government is focusing on the need to be open about uncertainty and to make the level of uncertainty clear when communicating with the public. This includes openness about any scientific uncertainty in the risk assessment and uncertainty about other factors in the risk management process.

6.13. Many government advisory committees deal with risk. When examining risk issues they may be confronted with scientific uncertainties. The Government accepts there is a need to ensure that advisory committees approach risk assessment more systematically and endorses the conclusions of the Chief Scientific Adviser, the Chief Medical Officer and the Chairman of the Food Standards Agency in their *"Review of Risk Procedures used by the Government's Advisory Committees dealing with Food Safety (July 2000)"* that a transparent and systematic risk assessment is the best way of approaching risk. This is particularly important where there is a lot of scientific uncertainty. This review, which involved CMOs in the devolved administrations, has been widely circulated to advisory committees, including non-food committees.

The Precautionary Approach

6.14. Where there is scientific uncertainty, the precautionary principle may be applied. This holds that absence of scientific proof should not delay or prevent proportionate measures to remove or reduce threats of serious harm. The Government is committed to taking a precautionary approach where appropriate. Government departments, working with the devolved administrations, are currently developing a UK approach. There are also international considerations; departments have contributed to European discussions and an EU Council Resolution on the precautionary principle was agreed in December 2000.

Cross-departmental working on risk issues

6.15. The Inquiry recommended that DH should be involved from the outset in all policy decisions involving risks to human health. Under a recent initiative departments are expected to apply Health Impact Assessments (HIA) to all new key policies. Departments are currently piloting a screening checklist to assess whether full HIAs are warranted.

6.16. The Inter-departmental Liaison Group on Risk Assessment (ILGRA), and its subgroup on risk communication, now ensure better sharing of information between government officials and a more consistent approach to risk across departments. ILGRA has promoted new collaborative approaches, fostered research on topics of cross-government relevance and provided a network for improving communication between those engaged in risk policy in different departments. ILGRA helps to avoid duplication of effort and promotes 'joined-up' thinking. One ILGRA initiative has been to help develop a cross-departmental approach to the application of the precautionary approach.

6.17. The Cabinet Office has a crucial role in central co-ordination on risk management. With ILGRA it attends the Treasury's Risk Management Steering Group. It also requires, and issues guidance on, Regulatory Impact Assessments.

Future Proposals

6.18. The Government accepts there is a need for further development in the way departments respond to situations of risk and uncertainty, and in the day to day working practices of officials working in policy areas. Issues of responsibility and accountability in food safety have been clarified by the creation of the FSA; in other areas further work may be needed. The position is clear in relation to financial accountability, but, at present, less so in relation to policy formulation and decision taking. Greater clarity would provide a firmer basis for timely action.

6.19. Responsibility for ensuring that risk assessment is properly carried out normally rests with the department with policy responsibility for that area. Scientific advisory committees may also be involved in organising and assessing such work.

6.20. It is more difficult to allocate responsibility for risk management decisions. The Treasury has been working on producing a broad framework for managing risk within which the specific issues of managing scientific risk would fit. The Treasury's *"Orange Book" – Management of Risk – A Strategic Overview January 2001* provides a generic model for addressing all risks to the achievement of an organisation's objectives. It sets out a life cycle for dealing with risk identification, assigning ownership, evaluation, assessing risk appetite, response to risk, gaining assurance and embedding review processes.

6.21. The "Orange Book" sets out the principles of good risk management. However, accountability and formal auditing of risk frameworks covering public health are complex. There might, therefore, be benefits to be gained from relevant departments developing and managing a structured system of responsibility specifically for risk management decisions that address public health. Such structures would not only help to focus individual departmental attention on risks to public health, but also ensure, within each department, transparency of process and quality management systems with which to monitor compliance.

6.22. The Government acknowledges that guidance alone in these areas will not be sufficient and that officials need to be thoroughly trained in its application. In addition to the programmes outlined in paragraphs 6.8. and 6.9., it is proposed to organise a workshop in summer 2001 for officials from across Government departments and agencies and devolved administrations to consider where improvements can be made in the handling of risk and uncertainty.

invitation?

6.23. The Government wants to develop a more robust and effective means of dealing with risk and uncertainty in public policy and is therefore working to produce its Statement on Risk, which will be put out to consultation.

6.24. **However, the Government is particularly interested in how risk management in the particular areas with which the Inquiry was concerned should best be addressed. It therefore seeks views on:**

- (i) (1) **Whether there are benefits from departments developing and managing a more structured system of responsibility for risk management decisions that relate to public health. If so, how might such systems be audited?**

- (ii) (2) **Whether the Government takes sufficient account of decision-making procedures that are used in the private sector to cover risk and uncertainty in these areas.**

- (iii) (3) **How the Government might best develop guidance on contingency planning and for assessing policy options.**

- (iv) (4) **Whether Government departments might add to their existing use of the Internet to provide information about the work of their advisory committees to invite public contribution and comment on risk issues.**

- (v) (5) **Ways of ensuring transparency of the process that departments use to take risk-based decisions.**

- (vi) (6) **How best to communicate low risk, when there is uncertainty associated with the assessment.**

6.25. **Are the answers to these questions any different for the devolved administrations?**

CHAPTER 7 – GOOD GOVERNMENT

Findings of the Inquiry

7.1.   Many of the Inquiry's findings relate to how government – both at large, and at the level of individual officials – should conduct its business. Some of these lessons have been covered in earlier chapters. This chapter addresses others which apply across the whole of government:

- government should ensure that it works in a joined-up way, and shares information effectively;

- the devolved administrations (broadly as successors of the previous territorial departments) should be fully involved in the exchange of information and, where appropriate, the process of policy development, particularly in relation to agreeing EU policy objectives;

- administrative barriers should not get in the way of effective action to protect public health.

7.2.   These recommendations can be considered under the following broad headings:

- Thinking ahead;

- Sharing information & working together; and

- Working with devolved administrations.

The Government Position

7.3.   The Government acknowledges that the whole approach and behaviour of departments and individuals will need to change to ensure that the lessons identified by the Inquiry are properly absorbed and implemented.

7.4.   As noted elsewhere in this response, the structure of government has altered considerably in recent years. Devolved legislatures and administrations have been established in Scotland, Wales and Northern Ireland. The Food Standards Agency has been established as a UK-wide body with a distinctive presence and accountability arrangements in each devolved area, responsible for the protection of public health in relation to food and empowered to publish the advice it gives to Ministers.

Thinking ahead

7.5.   The Inquiry identified the need for standing arrangements which identified departments to take the lead in areas of public safety where problems might arise, and for effective co-ordination mechanisms to be in place.

7.6.   The Government agrees with this finding. A principal aim of the Government's response to potential problems involving risks to human health is to ensure that there is minimum delay before effective action can be taken. Establishing lead responsibilities and standing arrangements before crises occur – and doing so in consultation with the devolved administrations – means that all parties know in advance what their responsibilities are and where the areas of common action will lie. This has always been the approach with civil emergencies. It is now being followed, with the full involvement of the devolved administrations, in the development of contingency plans for dealing with the possibility of BSE being found in sheep.

Sharing information & working together

7.7.   The importance of sharing information and knowledge is one of the major themes of the Report, especially the need for joined-up working between officials, experts and the wider public.

7.8.   The Inquiry has reinforced the Government's strongly held view that better co-ordination and information sharing are vitally important in improving public services. The Modernising Government White Paper of March 1999 highlighted the need for policy making to be joined-up. It said:

> *"in general too little effort has gone into making sure that policies are devised and delivered in a consistent and effective way across institutional boundaries – for example between different government departments, and between central and local government."*

7.9.   Since the White Paper was published, there has been work in central government and elsewhere to ensure that the Modernising Government vision is implemented. A Cabinet Office report on Modernising Government said that:

> *"There seems to be a common recognition of the benefits of joining up and a genuine desire to approach cross-cutting work in a new way. Policy makers need more help, though, to identify when joining up is necessary and what form it can best take."*

7.10.   The Inquiry encouraged greater co-operation on food safety and animal health, at all levels, between professionals and administrators and across departments.

7.11.   Government departments, including departments within the devolved administrations, have been forging closer links to improve co-operation and consultation on matters of shared interest. Formal arrangements such as the National Zoonoses Group, chaired by the Chief Medical Officer and with members from DH, MAFF, the FSA and the devolved administrations, are supported by greater informal contact. The Secretariat for SEAC is now drawn from three departments – MAFF, DH and the FSA. Departments are committed to sharing relevant information and advice and making it widely available to consumers. This includes information and papers relating to:

●   the scientific advisory committees in which they have a shared interest (for example the Advisory Committee on Animal Feedingstuffs and the Scientific Advisory Committee on Nutrition);

●   the results of collaborative surveillance and research;

- enforcement information, for example the BSE Enforcement Bulletin.

7.12. The Government has published a number of administrative agreements between different parts of Whitehall and the devolved administrations, called concordats. These agreements set out arrangements for co-operation in relation to policy, science, openness and other matters. For example, MAFF has concordats with the FSA, the Scottish Executive, the National Assembly for Wales and three of the Research Councils. A concordat with DARD will be in place shortly.

7.13. **The Government will consider these findings in the context of the Modernising Government agenda and increasing joined-up work and policy development, and welcomes ideas on how best to achieve these objectives.**

Working with the devolved administrations

7.14. Communication with the devolved administrations is an important aspect of joined-up government. Devolution has introduced fundamental structural changes in the government of the UK. The Inquiry has been helpful in highlighting issues which need to be addressed to ensure good liaison between the administrations, producing effective policy outcomes which have resonance throughout the UK.

7.15. The devolved administrations in Scotland, Wales and Northern Ireland do not have identical powers. But in general they have responsibility for food safety, animal and human health matters within their own locality and are subject to scrutiny for the decisions they take by locally elected representatives. Devolution has therefore increased the degree of scrutiny operating within the UK as a whole in the policy areas considered by the Inquiry.

7.16. While health and food safety are devolved matters, the FSA is a UK-wide body. It therefore provides a common source of independent scientific expertise and advice through the activities of a series of independent scientific advisory committees which operate at UK level. Yet the FSA is structured in a way which makes it flexible enough to accommodate local differences where they arise. It is also well placed to ensure that the best advice and expertise is drawn from across the UK.

7.17. Not all areas under consideration by the Inquiry are devolved. Controls over medicines (human and veterinary) are carried out throughout Great Britain by the relevant competent authority (Medicines Control Agency and Veterinary Medicines Directorate respectively). Northern Ireland carries out its own inspections and enforcement work in close co-operation with the MCA and VMD. Controls over medical devices are carried out throughout the UK by the Medical Devices Agency. The State Veterinary Service covers Scotland and Wales as well as England.

Findings of the Inquiry

7.18. The Inquiry's main findings in relation to the devolved administrations are that:

- arrangements should be put in place to facilitate a synchronised approach throughout the UK to common problems; and

- that action within the UK to deal with disease should be uniform and synchronised.

7.19. The Inquiry's findings relate to policy development in a pre-devolutionary context. Much policy development in the field of animal and animal/human health takes place in an EU context. Formal arrangements have been put in place to promote a synchronised approach on these issues, but this cannot always be achieved as, for example, legislation is now subject to the available timetable in different legislatures, although generally timing of policy implementation will be similar. Equally, it is not appropriate in the light of devolution to expect uniform policy solutions to be developed across the UK. The logic of devolution is that administrations are able to develop policies that are tailored for local circumstances. Such differences should not be seen as divisive or unhelpful. Rather, they illustrate a strength since they lead to more sensitive local policy making. The Inquiry's praise for Northern Ireland's separate approach to the ruminant feed ban shows that variations in policy can produce good results.

7.20. Arrangements are nonetheless in place to promote a common awareness of issues across the UK. The Government and the devolved administrations have all agreed a Memorandum of Understanding which commits each administration to information sharing and co-operation on policy development. For example, work takes place across the UK under an overall Concordat on Health and Social Care.

7.21. To provide a common starting point in terms of policy development, relevant papers are copied between administrations, and open discussion takes place in the many groups where all parts of the UK are represented. Effective working relationships have been built up at official level, and the FSA structure provides for co-ordinated advice both to London and the devolved administrations, while allowing each administration to take into account the particular needs and circumstances of its area.

7.22. These arrangements allow wider lessons to be learned than if identical arrangements were in place across the UK. Close liaison between officials will allow lessons – positive and negative – to be identified. Where one administration leads on good practice others can measure themselves against that standard.

7.23. **The Government is committed to continual improvements in the mechanisms for co-ordinating work and sharing information with the devolved administrations. Comments and views on how this commitment can best be achieved are welcomed.**

Enforcement of Legislation

7.24. This section deals with the Inquiry's concerns about the effective implementation of legislation. There is a need to ensure that when legislation is proposed and drafted, sufficient attention is given to the manner and effectiveness of its enforcement.

7.25. The Government accepts the need for adequate and timely consultation with enforcement bodies, efforts to ensure that the purpose of the legislation is understood and regular monitoring of the effectiveness of legislation and the enforcement process – leading, if necessary, to a review of the legislation. The number of enforcement bodies that may be involved in particular areas may make this difficult.

7.26. **The Government is addressing these issues and seeks comments and proposals on the arrangements necessary to ensure that legislation can be properly enforced and its effectiveness monitored.**

Roles of the Chief Medical Officer and Chief Veterinary Officer

7.27. This section deals with the different responsibilities of these posts in relation to providing independent advice, to making such advice public and to the scope of such advice. There are four Chief Medical Officers: one each for England, Scotland, Wales and Northern Ireland. The CMO for England is also the Chief Medical Adviser to the UK Government. There are two Chief Veterinary Officers: one for England, Wales and Scotland and one for Northern Ireland.

Findings of the Inquiry

7.28. The majority of the Inquiry's findings relate to the CMO for England and the CVO for Great Britain. They are, however, pertinent to all the CMOs and CVOs as are the specific findings on their functions. The Inquiry suggested that the CMO and CVO should, like the Food Standards Agency, have the power to publish the advice they give to Ministers. It emphasised the need to ensure that the public's trust in the CMO, as a source of objective and authoritative advice on risks to health, should not be put at risk. The Inquiry also raised the need for the roles of the CMO and CVO to be clarified in relation to making public statements on zoonoses and potential zoonoses.

Present Position

7.29. The Government thinks it important that the CMO should be able to provide objective advice both to Ministers and the public. Much of the advice that the Government requests from the CMO is intended, from the outset, to be made public, particularly when it is a formal report on a key issue; it is therefore presented in a straightforward and open way and is published when it goes forward to Ministers. The CMO has the role of an objective adviser who is able, as occasion demands, both to publish this advice and to advise the public directly and personally through the media.

7.30. The CVO is also able to provide advice to the public, although for some of the time he may be addressing a more limited, agriculturally based audience. He may, however, also give the general public information and advice on veterinary matters and the control of animal diseases. The Government does not, at present, ask the CVO for formal advice for publication in the same way as it does the CMO. It now proposes that the CVO should in future advise the Government as a whole on veterinary matters and may be asked to provide advice for publication.

7.31. On zoonoses, the CVO's responsibility is to provide advice, information and policy input on the disease situation in animals and to advise on the extent to which animals or their products may pose a risk to the public. The CVO is therefore responsible for identifying hazards and contributing to risk assessment. The CMO, acting on risk assessment information, is responsible for advising whether there is a risk to the public. The CMO and CVO work together to provide advice to the public and ensure that the risk is eliminated or minimised. The National Zoonoses Group, which the CMO chairs, supported by other, less formal contact, helps to ensure a co-ordinated approach.

Future Proposals

7.32.   The importance of maintaining a position of objectivity and independence for these posts is appreciated both within Government and by the public. The role of the CMO in providing advice on public health makes it particularly important that this independence should be safeguarded. But such a position must be balanced against the significant benefits to be gained from these senior professional advisers being fully involved in policy development and management within their departments.

7.33.   The position of the CMOs in the devolved administrations now reflects the structural and constitutional changes that devolution has brought. The role of each CMO is developing separately, but they continue to operate in the context of a co-ordinated approach by all CMOs to public health matters.

7.34.   **The Government, and the devolved administrations, would be interested in how the public sees the role of the CMOs and CVOs, particularly in relation to their independence from the Government and the devolved administrations, in giving advice and guidance to the public.**

Meat and Livestock Commission

7.35.   The Meat & Livestock Commission will be responding to the points made about its organisation by the Inquiry. It has already demonstrated its commitment to greater openness by deciding to place minutes of its meetings on the internet. The Commission will also be clarifying the position of the consultants it employs. The Government welcomes these developments.

CHAPTER 8 – LEGISLATIVE FRAMEWORK

Introduction

8.1.   This chapter sets out the Government's preliminary comments on the concerns raised by the Inquiry about the legislative framework available to deal with hazards such as BSE. **Views are invited, especially on any perceived gaps in the powers available to the Government to respond urgently and proportionately to an apparent hazard to human or animal health.**

Findings of the Inquiry

8.2.   The Inquiry's findings in relation to the legislative framework are:

  ● *Where an animal disease is identified, which could be transmitted to animals or humans via a range of possible routes, powers under UK and European law which enable Ministers to order the slaughter of animals, and the destruction of animal tissues or anything which might carry infection, should not be restricted merely because it cannot be established as a reasonable probability, as opposed to a mere possibility:*

  i.   *that the disease is transmissible; or*

  ii.   *that a particular animal may be infected by the disease in question; or*

  iii. *that particular organs or tissues in an animal may carry infection.*

  ● *Similarly, any powers under UK and European law which enable Ministers to adopt an alternative approach of banning the use of any substances for particular purposes in order to protection human or animal health should not be restricted merely because one or more of the matters referred to above cannot be established as a reasonable probability, as opposed to a mere possibility.*

  ● *Current medicines and consumer protection legislation should be reviewed with a view to giving the Government power to act swiftly and comprehensively to ban the use of any substances or processes which might pose a risk to human or animal health.*

  ● *The Government should review and clarify its powers under European law to introduce emergency measures for the protection of public and animal health in relation to outbreaks of disease where measures have previously been taken by the European Commission.*

8.3.   Two general concerns seem to underpin these findings:

  (a)   the availability of domestic emergency powers, provided by or permitted within the Community legal framework to protect public and animal health against risks associated with outbreaks of disease; and

  (b)   the Government's ability to exercise such available legal powers when the danger identified cannot be established as a probability as opposed to a mere possibility i.e. to reflect a precautionary approach to emergency legal powers.

Availability of Emergency Powers

8.4. The Government does not believe there are any serious gaps in its powers to take proportionate emergency action against hazards to human or animal health in relation to animals and animal products and food. **If, however, others are concerned about the scope of powers available to the Government in these circumstances, their views would be welcome.**

8.5. There are Community rules for the protection of animal and public health and food safety (Council Directives 89/662/EEC and 90/425/EEC). In relation to intra-community trade in animal products and live animals these expressly allow exceptional measures to be taken by Member States of origin and of destination in response to an outbreak of disease, zoonosis or other cause likely to cause a serious hazard to animals or to human health.

8.6. Where the outbreak is in the Member State of origin it is required to implement "the control or precautionary measures provided for in Community rules . . . or adopt any other measure which it deems appropriate". A Member State into which the relevant products are exported "may, on serious public or animal health grounds, take interim protective measures with regard to the establishments concerned". These measures are subject to Community review.

8.7. The existing harmonised Community rules which safeguard public and animal health at Community level therefore permit appropriate national controls in respect of new outbreaks or where new hazards arise which were not contemplated by existing Community measures.

8.8. There is also the desirability of achieving or safeguarding such national discretion when Community legislation is being negotiated. As a case in point, the European Commission's latest proposal for a Community Regulation laying down general principles of Food Law, establishing the European Food Authority and laying down procedures in matters of food safety, does contain emergency safeguard provisions enabling the Commission or Member States to take protective measures on an interim basis where it is found that existing controls are inadequate to protect consumers.

8.9. The Inquiry also expressed particular concern about the availability of powers to act comprehensively and swiftly in relation to medicines and generally under consumer protection legislation.

8.10. The approach to medicine regulation is fundamentally different from the approach to the regulation of food. It is a statutory system founded in EU law and based on prior authorisation before release of an individual medicinal product onto the market and appropriate pharmacovigilance measures. All such medicines have to meet a safety test which means that medicines for human and veterinary use cannot be marketed if they are harmful under normal conditions of use.

8.11. Medicines can be removed from the market by revocation or suspension of their marketing authorisation if they are found to be harmful. Such suspension can take place with immediate effect if it appears necessary to Ministers to do so in the interests of public safety. Suspension may ultimately lead to the withdrawal or variation of the marketing authorisation. Action is normally taken in respect of a specific product, but has been taken in relation to a particular group of products.

8.12. The Cosmetics Products (Safety) Regulations 1996 regulate substances used in cosmetics manufacture. DTI has the powers to act swiftly if concerns arise on the safety of cosmetics ingredients. DTI and DoH agree on the need for better liaison between departments to enable both to act quickly and effectively with regard to medicines and consumer protection legislation. These departments are working together to improve communication.

8.13. The Medical Devices Regulations 1994 regulate medical devices containing substances or material derived from animal origin. The Regulations include safeguard clauses which allow the Secretary of State to remove devices from the market quickly, by means of Notices under the Consumer Protection Act, if there are concerns over public health or safety.

Exercise of Powers in Uncertainty

8.14. The Inquiry considers it desirable that 'legislation should clearly empower Ministers to take precautionary measures in a situation where the existence of a hazard is uncertain' and that 'there are areas where this may not be the case'.

8.15. The Government believes that in all reasonably foreseeable circumstances it will have the legal powers to act proportionately to take protective measures in response to new hazards, even where they are uncertain. It recognises that, depending on the domestic or Community legal instrument applicable to the particular case, the availability of powers may depend on an express Ministerial judgement (for example as to the presence of a disease, or the prospect of a hazard to human health), rather than providing unfettered freedom to act at Government discretion. Such constraints reflect the intentions of Parliament (or, as the case may be, Community legislative institutions in which the Government has participated) at the time.

8.16. It is worth noting that even where there is no such express requirement in the directly relevant legislation, the exercise of powers will be subject to obligations on Government to act in accordance with the law and the principles of good administration, taking account of the human rights of all parties potentially affected. In cases of uncertainty, these obligations can assume particular importance; but they should not be incompatible with proportionate precautionary action against a potentially serious, if uncertain, hazard.

8.17. **The Government is interested in circumstances in which others believe that the relevant domestic or EU provisions do not provide for it to address the possibility, though not necessarily likelihood, of a serious hazard.**

Devolved Legislation

8.18. The new constitutional balance introduced by devolution may lead to greater divergence between the powers applicable in different parts of the United Kingdom. However, the desirability of achieving a high level of consistency is recognised, particularly in regard to shared public health hazards and the implementation of Community obligations. To achieve that end the devolved administrations continue to work closely with relevant Whitehall departments and each other, through communication and consultation.

CHAPTER 9 – SUMMARY OF ISSUES FOR CONSULTATION

This Chapter brings together all the invitations to express views and contribute ideas that appear in this Response.

Science and Government

The Government welcomes views on what else might be done to ensure that departments maintain an effective research management and scientific advisory system. (4.11.)

The Government wants to continue to develop arrangements to ensure that the full range of scientific opinions can be heard by those developing policy and would be interested in views on how this might best be undertaken. (4.17.)

The Government would welcome views on the arrangements for research management in Chapter 4 and on whether there are different approaches that might be tested to ensure that the high quality research necessary to inform and evaluate government policy can be procured. (4.21.)

The Government would welcome views on whether the proposed arrangements for the development and publication of research strategies are likely to be sufficient for external observers to identify gaps and recognise priorities in departmental research programmes. (4.25.)

The Government would welcome views on whether a website providing access to information about publicly-funded R&D programmes and projects should be available and, if so, what the priorities should be as to its contents. (4.26.)

The Government already undertakes some "horizon scanning" for possible risks. What other approaches to identifying potential risks would be useful? (4.31.)

The Government is strengthening its research co-ordination arrangements. Are there any other approaches to this that it could adopt? (4.36.)

The Government and the devolved administrations would be interested in views on whether the answers to the questions posed in this chapter are different in relation to Scotland, Wales or Northern Ireland. (4.2.)

Openness

The Government is interested to know whether the initiatives by the FSA in this chapter meet the challenges of public confidence in food safety and the specific lessons of BSE. Is there more that the FSA might do? (5.12.)

How might departments best implement the Government's commitment to trusting the public and continue to develop ways of being open and consulting widely while developing policy? (5.18.)

The Government is interested in views on the effectiveness of the steps it is taking to be more open and so generate greater public trust in its handling of food safety issues. In particular:

- does the programme of action described in this chapter meet the need for greater openness identified by the Inquiry?

- should government departments do more to secure public trust through greater openness on food safety and related issues and, if so, what in particular should they be doing? (5.22.)

Risk and Uncertainty

The Government is particularly interested in how risk management in the particular areas with which the Inquiry was concerned, in science and in food safety, should best be addressed. It therefore seeks views on:

- Whether there are benefits from departments developing and managing a more structured system of responsibility for risk management decisions that relate to public health. If so, how might such systems be audited?

- Whether the Government takes sufficient account of decision-making procedures that are used in the private sector to cover risk and uncertainty in these areas.

- How the Government might best develop guidance on contingency planning and for assessing policy options.

- Whether government departments might add to their existing use of the Internet to provide information about the work of their advisory committees to invite public contribution and comment on risk issues.

- Ways of ensuring transparency of the process that departments use to take risk-based decisions.

- How best to communicate low risk when there is uncertainty associated with the assessment. (6.24.)

Are the answers to these questions any different for the devolved administrations? (6.25.)

Good Government

The Government will consider findings set out in Chapter 7 in the context of the Modernising Government agenda and increasing joined-up work and policy development, and welcomes ideas on how best to achieve these objectives. (7.13.)

The Government is committed to continual improvements in the mechanisms for co-ordinating work and sharing information with the devolved administrations. Comments and views on how this commitment can best be achieved are welcomed. (7.23.)

The Government is addressing these issues and seeks comments and proposals on the arrangements necessary to ensure that legislation can be properly enforced and its effectiveness monitored. (7.26.)

The Government, and the devolved administrations, would be interested in how the public sees the role of the CMOs and CVOs, particularly in relation to their independence from the Government and devolved administrations in giving advice and guidance to the public. (7.34.)

Legislative Framework

Views are invited, especially on any perceived gaps in the powers available to the Government to respond urgently and proportionately to an apparent hazard to human or animal health. (8.1.)

If, however, others are concerned about the scope of powers available to the Government in these circumstances, their views and proposals would be welcome. (8.4.)

The Government is interested in circumstances in which others believe that the relevant domestic or EU provisions do not provide for it to address the possibility, though not necessarily likelihood, of a serious hazard. (8.17.)

DETAILED FINDINGS

1.   This annex presents the 167 detailed findings contained in the BSE Inquiry Report. It explains the Government's position on each of these findings, setting out what action has already been taken, what is planned and how others will be involved in the final outcome.

2.   Most of the findings are drawn from Volume 1 of the Report where the Inquiry sets out its "Findings and Conclusions" (see Chapter 14, "Lessons to be learned"). Others have been taken from Volumes 2 to 9 and Volume 11, which cover the Inquiry's detailed analysis of events from the BSE story.

2.   The Inquiry's individual findings have been brought together in this annex under broad subject headings. In every case there is a reference to the relevant part of the Inquiry Report. The areas covered are:

    (a)   the nature of TSEs (pages 40-42);

    (b)   disease control (pages 43-45);

    (c)   relations between Government Departments (pages 46-48);

    (d)   enforcement (page 49);

    (e)   devolved administrations (pages 50-56);

    (f)   medicines (pages 57-63);

    (g)   non-food routes of infection (pages 64-67);

    (h)   research (pages 68-69);

    (i)   advisory committees (pages 70-75);

    (j)   risk management and communication (pages 76-78);

    (k)   legislation (pages 79-80); and,

    (l)   variant CJD (pages 81-83).

4.   The Government would welcome views on all these findings, and on the way forward.

THE NATURE OF TSES

Finding	Response
1. TSEs may occur in species in which they have previously been unknown (Volume 1, para. 1264).	It is possible that TSEs will be identified in species in which they have previously been unknown, whether sporadically or by inter-species transmission. The Minister of Agriculture, Fisheries and Food and the Secretary of State for Health have therefore asked Professor Horn to lead a small team of scientists in reviewing the current state of understanding of the origin of BSE in cattle. In doing so they will take into account the scientific and epidemiological evidence presented to the Inquiry, the findings of a Working Group of the EU Scientific Steering Committee, which is also looking into this matter, and other ongoing work in the UK and elsewhere.
2. It is possible that TSEs develop sporadically in other animal species as they do in humans (Volume 1, para. 1264).	
3. If TSEs develop sporadically and rarely in farm animals, as they do in humans, they may well pass undetected. This is particularly the case where farm animals are slaughtered for consumption when young and thus before clinical signs normally develop (Volume 1, para. 1264).	The Government accept that TSEs may pass undetected in young, pre-clinical animals. With respect to BSE in cattle the control measures now in place take account of this possibility and have significantly reduced the risk of infected cattle entering the human food chain. Limited precautionary measures have also been taken in respect of the possibility of BSE in sheep and goats. However, this does not remove the possibility of infected animals from other species passing undetected. The most effective way of reducing this risk would be to have a diagnostic test which would be sensitive enough to detect infected animals in the pre-clinical stages and could be used in widespread screening programmes. More than one test may be required given the variety of strains and species in farm animals. Government is increasing its efforts to encourage development of such tests. Through the Joint Funders Group a meeting to encourage collaboration between academics and small biotechnology companies has been arranged for February 2001. This will presage a new call for research proposals on diagnostic development for which the funders have allocated research funding.
4. TSEs may be transmissible between the same species and between different species (Volume 1, para. 1265).	The Government agrees with these findings. The controls in place recognise the danger of intraspecies recycling and the possibility of transmitting TSEs from one species to another. Since 1996 meat and bone meal derived from ruminants has been prohibited from inclusion in animal feed of all domestic food species. The controls have recently been reviewed by the Food Standards Agency. The Agency concluded that they provided effective risk reduction and that they should remain in place.
5. TSEs may be transmissible within animal feed and human food (Volume 1, para. 1265)	
6. Tissues in an animal incubating a TSE may be infectious before the animal has developed clinical signs of the disease (Volume 1, para. 1265).	The Government agrees with this finding. Ongoing pathogenesis studies in both sheep and cattle are providing valuable data on which tissues become infected at which stage of disease development in the animal. This will help further to identify the risks from infectivity coming from pre-clinical animals. See also comments in relation to finding 3.

Finding	Response
7. It is possible to distinguish between the level of infectivity, or titre, likely to be found in the different tissues of an animal incubating a TSE. The brain and spinal cord, in the later stages of incubation, are the highest risk tissues (Volume 1, para. 1265).	Current Specified Risk Material (SRM) controls are designed to prevent all high risk tissues from cattle from entering the human food chain. Ongoing research is further developing our knowledge of the distribution of infectivity in the tissues of sheep of different genotype. SEAC has recommended that further work should be undertaken on pigs and poultry to establish whether they can be carriers of disease even if they do not show clinical signs of disease.
8. A very small quantity of infective material may be sufficient to transmit a TSE by the oral route (Volume 1, para. 1265).	Data from attack rate experiments have shown that this is the case.
9. Risk of oral transmission of a TSE will be greatly reduced if high risk tissues are removed from the food chain (Volume 1, para. 1265).	The Government agrees with this finding. Legislation prohibiting the inclusion of Specified Risk Material (SRM) was first introduced for cattle in 1989 and for sheep and goats in 1996. The controls in place have been regularly reviewed and the legislation strengthened as new scientific information has emerged. The latest review was undertaken by the Food Standards Agency and was published in December 2000. Their conclusion was that there should be no immediate change in the SRM rules, but that these should be kept under review. Future changes may depend on the development of diagnostic tests that could indicate whether TSE infection was present in carcasses or in the live animal in the pre-clinical stage.

Wider Community SRM controls, banning intestines from cattle of all ages, were formally adopted by the Commission in December 2000. Legislation is already in place in the UK. |
| 10. The process of rendering animal parts to produce MBM which is then incorporated in animal feed, will result in the pooling of material from many animals and the wide dissemination of infection from a single infective animal (Volume 1, para. 1266).

11. The rendering process cannot be relied upon to inactivate TSEs (Volume 1, para. 1266). | The Government agrees with these findings. That is why controls have been put in place and strengthened over time to prevent further infection and to stop the spread of the BSE agent. Research investigating how well different rendering procedures inactivate TSE infectivity has shown that some procedures fail to inactivate TSEs in rendered material. BSE is particularly resistant to inactivation procedures. |
| 12. Recycling animal protein carries a greater risk of spreading infection with a TSE where it is carried out within the same species (Volume 1, para. 1266). | Empirical evidence would suggest that this is true. However, insufficient is known about the nature of the species barrier to be certain that it is always the case. |

Finding	Response
13. Recycling animal protein carries a greater risk of spreading infection with a TSE where the protein is derived from high risk tissue (Volume 1, para. 1266).	Controls on the use of SRM in animal feed, introduced in 1990 and strengthened subsequently, address the point. These need to be kept under review as new information becomes available. Ongoing pathogenesis studies will tell us more about the stage of incubation at which different tissues become infective. New tests may also be developed which allow PrP^{Sc} or some other marker of infection to be detected in carcass tissues or at the pre-clinical phase in the live animal.
14. Where a TSE has a lengthy incubation period, recycling may spread the disease very widely before its emergence is detected (Volume 1, para. 1266).	The Government accepts this finding. See comments for findings 1-3 and 6.
15. While it is reasonable in . . . 1989 to accept the hypothesis that the cases of BSE being reported had come about through the rendering of carcasses of sheep infected with extant strains of scrapie established in the national flock, this theory is no longer plausible . . . The cause . . . is likely to have been a new prion mutation in cattle, or possibly sheep . . . other mammalian species whose carcass waste was included in MBM cannot be excluded. It is conceivable that the conversion of normal prion protein into its infective form was initiated not by a gene mutation, but by an environmental agent, such as a toxic chemical; this has not yet been achieved experimentally. Current knowledge suggests that the original agent was not the unmodified scrapie agent or agents. It is now not possible to be sure which of the hypotheses as to the origin of the novel agent is correct (Volume 2, para. 7.3).	The origin of BSE in cattle remains uncertain and is a matter of considerable public interest. The Minister of Agriculture, Fisheries and Food and the Secretary of State for Health have therefore asked Professor Horn to lead a small team of scientists in reviewing the current state of understanding of the origin. In doing so they will take into account the scientific and epidemiological evidence presented to the Inquiry, the findings of a Working Group of the EU Scientific Steering Committee, which is also looking into this matter, and other ongoing work in the UK and elsewhere.

DISEASE CONTROL

Finding	Response
16. An effective system of animal disease surveillance is a prerequisite to the effective control of animal diseases (Volume 1, para. 1268).	The Government supports this finding. The ongoing Review of Veterinary Surveillance in England and Wales will help to strengthen the surveillance systems which are already in place. Scotland and Northern Ireland are fully involved in discussing the Review and will address the issues of animal disease surveillance raised as they affect those parts of the UK.
17. An effective system of passive surveillance will depend upon farmers and their veterinarians having the incentive and the facility for drawing instances of animal disease to the attention of the State Veterinary Service (Volume 1, para. 1268).	Farmers and veterinarians have a key role in passive surveillance. The above Review provides an opportunity to consider how to engage them more effectively and to look at questions about access to Veterinary Investigation Centres (VICs) and their equivalents in Scotland and Northern Ireland.
18. Research into methods of diagnosis should form an integral part of an animal disease surveillance system (Volume 1, para. 1268).	A diagnostic test development programme has been instituted as part of MAFF's veterinary surveillance function. See also comments for finding 3.
19. The proximity of the nearest veterinary centre of investigation to the farm where the disease occurs will be an important factor in determining whether or not a casualty is referred for pathological examination (Volume 1, para. 1268).	
20. The identification of BSE demonstrated the importance of the animal disease surveillance system of the State Veterinary Service and of the close links that existed between the VICs and the CVL (Volume 1, para. 1268).	The Government agrees with this finding. The Veterinary Investigation Centres (VICs) and the Central Veterinary Laboratory (CVL) have now been brought together in a single Agency – the Veterinary Laboratories Agency. This has helped to strengthen internal communications even further. There is also close liaison between the VLA and the Scottish Agricultural College, which provides animal disease surveillance in Scotland.

Finding	Response
21. It is important that details of a new disease which may have implications for human and animal health should be disseminated within the State and private veterinary systems in order to encourage the reporting of similar cases (Volume 1, para. 1268).	The National Zoonoses Group, chaired by the CMO, is a joint DH / MAFF Group attended by the HSE, FSA and the devolved administrations. The Group includes experts from the PHLS, VLA and representatives from the Local Government Co-ordinating Body (LACOTS). This Group is responsible for managing the risks to human health posed by zoonoses and also considers new and emerging diseases or syndromes. A summary of the main topics discussed and the decisions reached at Group meetings are available to the public and to private veterinarians on the internet. In addition, information about any new diseases that may have an impact for animal health are notified to the *Veterinary Record*, a publication with a wide readership amongst the veterinary community. Further consideration will be given to this issue in connection with the ongoing Review of Veterinary Surveillance in England and Wales.
22. Lead responsibility must be clearly established for co-ordinating the scientific response to a new disease or a new outbreak of disease (Volume 1, para. 1269).	Agreed. The "Guidelines 2000" on scientific advice and policy making, re-issued by the Office of Science and Technology in July 2000, make clear that Government Departments: "should ensure they have mechanisms in place for early identification of issues which affect more than one department or agency. Departments should involve the Office of Science and Technology in all substantive or sensitive issues which cross departmental boundaries." See also comments for finding 87.
23. Provision should be made for training veterinarians in epidemiology. Joint postgraduate training programmes in epidemiology for trainees in veterinary medicine and public health medicine should be encouraged (Volume 1, para. 1272).	The need for an effective veterinary epidemiology resource is recognised and is being considered as part of the ongoing Review of Veterinary Surveillance in England and Wales. The Epidemiology Department at VLA now comprises the largest group of post graduate trained veterinary epidemiologists (13) in the world. Competitive tendering for research contracts ensures that other sources of expertise can be employed. Government advisory committees routinely employ specialist epidemiologists. See also comments on finding 37.

Views of interested parties are invited on the question of joint training for veterinarians and public health specialists. |
| 24. Epidemiologists, particularly those in the public sector, should make available the data upon which their conclusions are based (Volume 1, para. 1272). | The Government accepts this finding. Release of data by Departments to the scientific community is covered in the "Guidelines 2000", published by the Office of Science and Technology in July last year. |

Finding	Response
25. We urge those whose task it is to answer these questions about the strengths and weaknesses of passive surveillance not to lose sight of the importance of an effective early warning system for an outbreak of a disease such as BSE, and of the corresponding need to encourage referral of cases by individual farmers and veterinarians (Volume 2, para. 7.75).	The Government recognises the force of these findings. One of the primary objectives of veterinary surveillance is rapidly to detect new diseases, infections and intoxications of livestock via an effective early warning system. This requires the availability, and take up by farmers and veterinarians, of diagnostic tests. These issues are being considered as part of the ongoing Review of Veterinary Surveillance in England and Wales. They are also being considered in Scotland and Northern Ireland. See findings 17-19 above.
26. We recognise the cost implications of maintaining the current network of laboratories, let alone providing more diagnostic tests more cheaply or freely in order to encourage submissions. It is unlikely that even a free service would ensure the submission of 100 per cent of cases that with hindsight turned out to be informative or significant. What is important is that some systematic assessment is made of the costs and benefits of the different approaches, such as targets for representative submissions, facilitated by vouchers or discounts, or agreements with sentinel veterinary practices, or other options. Economic realities mean that some form of subsidy needs to be considered if the cost:benefit ratio is to be swung in favour of specimen submission (Volume 2, paras. 7.67-7.77).	

RELATIONS BETWEEN GOVERNMENT DEPARTMENTS

Finding	Response
27. Collaboration between MAFF and DH, and between CVO and CMO, must be maintained in considering the potential for animal diseases to threaten human health and the steps that should be taken in response to any potential zoonosis. Consideration should be given to whether a formal structure is the best means of achieving this (Volume 1, para. 1269).	Agreed. The need for better co-operation has been addressed through the formation of the National Zoonoses Group, chaired by the Chief Medical Officer, which addresses the risks to human health posed by zoonoses and also considers new and emerging diseases. Meetings of the Group are attended by DH, MAFF, HSE, FSA, the devolved administrations, VLA and the PHLS. And the Surveillance Group for Diseases and Infections in Animals, chaired by the Chief Veterinary Officer, includes members drawn from DH, FSA, PHLS, VLA and the devolved administrations. This Group looks at information on animal diseases, including new and emerging diseases. Ways of further improving the relationship between the CVO and UK CMOs will be looked at specifically by the National Zoonoses Group.
28. Where animal or public health is at stake, resort should be had to the best source of scientific advice, wherever it is to be found, without delay (Volume 1, para. 1269).	Agreed. The Office of Science and Technology's "Guidelines 2000" cover the need for Departments to ensure that they have the capacity to recognise and to react quickly and efficiently to new issues. And they emphasise the importance of assembling all relevant scientific disciplines necessary to address the problem, drawing on the best expert sources, both within and outside Government.
29. Advantage should be taken of the expertise and resources of the PHLS whenever the possibility of a potential zoonosis exists (Volume 1, para. 1269).	Agreed. The PHLS is represented on key interdepartmental groups, including the National Zoonoses Group, the Advisory Committee on Dangerous Pathogens and the Surveillance Group for Animal Infections, which helps to promote effective collaboration. There is a formal Memorandum of Understanding between VLA and PHLS.
30. The activities of the MLC in the period up to 20 March 1996 do not appear to have represented all its statutory objectives. The MLC has submitted to us proposals in relation to its future role. We recommend that these receive consideration in the light of our report (Volume 1, para. 1302).	The MLC will be putting proposals to Ministers shortly, aimed at achieving a better balance between its responsibilities to different stakeholders, particularly consumers. These proposals will be carefully considered.

Finding	Response
31. The BSE story illustrates the importance of the agencies dealing with human health and those dealing with animal health working together if threats to human health posed by zoonoses or potential zoonoses are to be managed in the most effective way (Volume 2, para. 7.79).	The Government agrees with these findings. See also findings 27 and 29.
32. By way of example, there are a number of respects in which the PHLS might have been able to offer MAFF assistance in relation to BSE (Volume 2, para. 7.82).	
33. We reiterate the importance of continuing to develop closer collaboration in the investigation and management of human and animal disease (Volume 2, para. 7.82).	
34. What matters equally is that administrators, vets, physicians and others recognise the importance of alerting each other to new potential zoonoses. (Volume 2, para. 7.83).	The Government agrees that an effective flow of information must occur. At central government level this is achieved through the National Zoonoses Group and the Surveillance Group for Diseases and Infections in Animals. Public Health Liaison Groups have been established at the local level to discuss animal diseases and infections which may pose a risk to human health; these include representatives from the PHLS, VLA Regional Laboratories, the Communicable Disease Surveillance Centre and the devolved administrations.
35. The BSE story suggests to us that such collaboration may be facilitated by clear allocation of a lead responsibility for a new disease, or a new outbreak of disease, to an organisation and, within that, to an individual who will need to consider which other organisations need to be involved (Volume 2, para. 7.83).	The Government accepts this finding in principle and will consider what further action might be necessary.

Finding	Response
36. We think that the BSE story also suggests that consideration should be given to joint working at a more detailed level, especially where there is very limited specialist expertise. For example, there could be practical advantages in combining what are currently separate VLA and PHLS laboratories which may work on sub-typing the same organism (Volume 2, para. 7.84).	The Government endorses the need for close working between VLA and PHLS. The laboratories already have a formal Memorandum of Understanding aimed at maximising shared knowledge, facilities and capabilities to meet the national need. There is close integration of services, common databases, standard methodologies and complementary work programmes. Where appropriate, common facilities are used, e.g. for typing and reference services. Joint reference services are already provided for brucellosis, botulism and rabies. The scope for collaboration on other diseases and on research and surveillance projects is regularly considered; e.g. the laboratories recently collaborated on an abattoir survey of pigs, looking for salmonella and other food-borne zoonotic pathogens.
37. Similarly consideration should be given to whether two separate organisations are needed to study the epidemiology of a disease which affects both animals and humans. A number of those giving evidence to the Inquiry commented on the lack of veterinary epidemiologists in the UK. Yet, as we said above, the methodologies used by epidemiologists in human and animal disease are essentially the same (Volume 2, para. 7.84).	Both the Department of Health and MAFF will continue to have need of access to specialist epidemiological expertise; on the one hand for human diseases (not all of which derive from animals), and on the other for animal diseases (not all of which affect humans). The need for close collaboration on the epidemiology of zoonoses is acknowledged above.
	The shortage of veterinary epidemiologists has been addressed in several ways. Links have been developed with the University of Massey in New Zealand, significantly increasing the number of veterinary epidemiologists available to the VLA. MAFF has also funded a five year fellowship in Veterinary Epidemiology at Liverpool University and members of the VLA Epidemiology Department have designed and run an MSc course in conjunction with colleagues at the London School of Hygiene and Tropical Medicine and the Royal Veterinary College. Additionally, the team within the VLA Epidemiology Department has been significantly expanded through a strategic recruiting and training programme, bringing a range of expertise to bear on epidemiological analyses. The suggestion that all epidemiologists use the same methodologies overlooks the range of different knowledge and skills required to operate effectively within either the veterinary or medical fields. See also finding 23.
38. Establishing before a crisis arises where lead responsibility for advice lies is highly desirable. While HSE has overall responsibility for occupational safety guidance and the consistency and principles of the approach to this, we see no reason why Departments should not under standing arrangements take the lead on some matters (Volume 6, para. 8.232).	The Government agrees with this recommendation and will consider what further action might be necessary. The Government has already established the FSA to take the lead on all food safety issues.

ENFORCEMENT

39. When Regulations that have implications for human or animal health fall to be enforced by local authorities: clear guidance should be given to the local authorities as to the importance of the Regulations and the manner of their enforcement; there should be statutory provision enabling central government to monitor the standards of compliance and enforcement (Volume 1, para. 1277).

This is done already. In relation to food, the statutory provisions are set out in the Food Standards Act 1999 (Sections 12-16). The Food Standards Agency now has a Framework Agreement with local authorities which covers both guidance and monitoring. The Agency's internal guidance helps to ensure that local authority enforcement aspects are fully considered in all proposed regulations.

With regard to animal health legislation, GB Agriculture Ministers have the power to ensure that local authorities carry out their duty of enforcement under Section 59 of the Animal Health Act 1981. Where secondary legislation is made under the European Community Act, the normal practice is to include equivalent provisions where the local authority is the enforcement authority. Guidance is given to local authorities wherever necessary. Broadly similar arrangements apply in Northern Ireland.

A new best value performance indicator to apply from April 2001, developed by the Food Standards Agency, Health and Safety Executive, and relevant Government departments, measures the performance of local authorities in respect of Environmental Health and Trading Standards. Authorities' performance will be measured on their adherence to and monitoring of their enforcement policies and procedures, and risk-based inspection programmes. Annually, authorities must publish their scores and targets for improvement in performance plans. In England and Wales, these are audited by the Audit Commission, and results published nationally. If an authority is found to be failing in its duty of best value, recommendations can be made to the Secretary of State for the Environment, Transport and the Regions (for England), or the relevant Minister at the National Assembly for Wales, for intervention to be made. Intervention could range from an authority being directed to amend their plans, to, at worst, the removal of responsibility for the function from an authority altogether. Similar indicators and arrangements apply in Scotland and Wales, although Scottish authorities report on a voluntary basis.

40. Measures that depend on particular slaughterhouse procedures being followed need to be based on informed understanding of practical working conditions (Volume 1, para. 1277).

The Government accepts this recommendation. The Food Standards Agency will ensure that all such measures are informed by the experience of Meat Hygiene Service or DARD Veterinary Service staff working in slaughterhouses. Consultation with slaughterhouse operators is now normal practice.

41. Government Departments should clearly tell both the public and those responsible for enforcement the reasons for, and the importance of, any precautionary measures that they introduce (Volume 1, para. 1278).

Agreed. The FSA's standard operating procedures, debating issues publicly and consulting stakeholders, should ensure a climate in which both the public and those involved with implementation are clear about the need for any new measure. Formal links between the FSA and the Meat Hygiene Service, DARD Veterinary Service and local authorities are already helping to facilitate clear communication on food law enforcement.

DEVOLVED ADMINISTRATIONS

42. Arrangements need to be in place which will facilitate a synchronised approach throughout the United Kingdom to common problems of animal health, or animal and human health (Volume 1, para. 1282).

The Government accepts these recommendations. The Government and the devolved administrations already work closely together on matters of animal and human health, as in other areas. Devolution means that while policy discussions are carried out in a synchronised way, implementation can be tuned to the particular needs of each of the four administrations.

43. It will normally be desirable that action taken within the United Kingdom to deal with disease should be uniform and synchronized (Volume 1, para. 1289).

Many discussions on animal and animal/human health take place in the context of a common EU framework. Concordats are being put in place covering both health and agriculture, which will provide an effective framework, allowing the four UK administrations to work closely together. Each administration is committed to the sharing of information and to co-operating on policy development.

44. So far as animal diseases, particularly those which may involve risk to human health, are concerned, a clear understanding should exist as to: the identification of those areas where a uniform and synchronized policy and/or implementation is required and who is to take the lead; the sharing of resources and information; a structure for consultation and joint decision-making that minimises unnecessary delay (Volume 1, para. 1289).

The State Veterinary Service is a shared resource across Great Britain, and is paralleled in Northern Ireland by the DARD Veterinary Service. The Food Standards Agency is accountable to all four UK administrations. The establishment of the Agency is a significant step towards addressing the Inquiry's concerns.

Finding	Response
45. [On] the incidence of the disease, it is only now that apparent problems over the confidentiality of the GB data collected by Mr Wilesmith of CVL have been overcome . . . allowing fuller epidemiological analysis of the evolution of the disease. That has offered new insights about the pattern and thus the genesis and means of spread of BSE. We were not told of any similar analysis in Northern Ireland reviewing Mr Denny's work, but note that analysis of the data on DANI's [cattle-tracking] system might have fewer confidentiality difficulties than CVL perceived under the powers they used to log data in GB . . . all available 'regional' case studies should be used to the full to carry forward investigative work . . . such studies might also usefully pay particular attention to the 'island' experiences of the Channel Islands, the Isle of Man and the Scottish Islands, both . . . [on] the history of the disease and . . . the effects of local measures taken to arrest it (Volume 9, para. 16.43).	The Government agrees with this recommendation. A new anonymous database is now available, which facilitates freer access. The Veterinary Laboratories Agency has collaborated on this with Massey University (New Zealand) since 1996. Other datasets exist, though they may have confidentiality problems of their own. Under-reporting also needs to be taken into account when using any of these data. See also comments on finding 24.
46. In the case of the ruminant feed ban, the Northern Ireland administration did indeed form its own separate views . . . But this was the exception rather than the rule . . . We do not criticise this practice, which had the merit of economy of effort and consistency of advice . . . [and] reflected the fact that most of the available knowledge lay in Whitehall . . . it meant that although separately responsible, those Ministers and their officials were relying on the analysis provided for their counterparts in London rather than on independent advice in giving their approval to legislation. This issue is by no means restricted to BSE alone, and is beyond our remit to explore. We simply note that, so far as BSE was concerned, the exercise of the separate legislative powers was mainly rubber-stamping (Volume 9, paras 17.9-17.10).	The Government agrees that all four UK administrations should be able readily to draw on the same information and expert advice to inform decision-taking. Consideration will be given to placing the current arrangements on a more formal footing.

Finding	Response
47. We were particularly struck by the multidisciplinary approach of the Welsh Office Health Professionals Group and its integration of both epidemiological and environmental health advice. The Group's combined analysis bridged the gaps that existed nationally between those knowledgeable on epidemiological techniques, human health issues and the actual processes involved in slaughtering and butchery. Using its collective knowledge the Group identified some of the potential pathways of infection, points at which specific hazards needed to be addressed and enforcement monitored, and wider issues on which research and investigation were needed. It was in a position to make judgements about the application of the precautionary principle. The effectiveness of this arrangement was undoubtedly strengthened by the close association between the Welsh Office and the Public Health Laboratory Service (PHLS) . . . We believe this arrangement might usefully be considered elsewhere (Volume 9, paras. 17.33-17.34).	Agreed. Stronger interdisclipinary arrangements are already in place in all four administrations. Consideration will be given to how far this meets the Inquiry's concern.
48. We noted the role played by the Chief Scientific Officer in Northern Ireland as a team member generally and as an experienced analyst and adviser on food safety issues. This seemed to us to offer a model for consideration where policy development and assessment of risk are concerned (Volume 9, para. 17.35).	The Government accepts this finding. The Food Standards Agency is well placed to co-ordinate risk assessment advice for all parts of the UK on food safety matters.

Finding	Response
49. We believe that it was important for the Territorial Departments to have access to SEAC papers, but they needed to avoid being deluged with documents. One option would have been to circulate agendas and minutes and enable the territorial officials to call for papers that interested them. However, a perennial problem with this kind of arrangement is that it is not always obvious from a title on an agenda what the real subject matter or purpose of a paper is; indeed it may only become apparent during discussion at the meeting what really concerns the expert advisers. Even if all the papers had been circulated, the Territorial Departments might have found it difficult . . . to work out what was of significance for them. Despite these difficulties, more effective arrangements need to be in place that achieve the right balance between deluge and drought (Volume 9, para. 17.40).	The Government accepts this recommendation. SEAC now reports direct to Ministers in all four parts of the UK. Officials from the UK Health and Agriculture Departments and the Food Standards Agency work closely in relation to SEAC, routinely exchanging information and analyses to promote effective understanding of the Committee's activities.
50. As we note above, one of the benefits of greater sharing of information might have been that MAFF and DH would have been alerted to some of the very real concerns being felt by some of those working in the Territorial Departments. It seems to us that that in turn might have affected the urgency with which some matters – such as the importance of compliance with the SBO ban or the hazards inherent in methods of head-splitting and brain removal – were addressed and, if necessary, passed back to the experts for consideration. Arrangements which ensure feedback from the Territorial Departments to the officials assessing the risk and advising Ministers centrally, at the appropriate point in the policy-making cycle, would be valuable (Volume 9, para. 17.41).	The Government accepts this recommendation. Good links already exist between MAFF, DH and the devolved administrations in the areas of human and animal health. And the Food Standards Agency operates across the whole of the UK. The Government, together with the devolved administrations, will consider whether any further action might be necessary. The authorisation of medicines for human and veterinary use is carried out by the relevant authority (the Medicines Control Agency and the Veterinary Medicines Directorate respectively) for the whole of the UK. The MCA and VMD carry out inspection and enforcement visits on behalf of Scotland and Wales; Northern Ireland carries out its own visits in close co-operation with MCA. All four administrations recognise that maintaining a UK-wide strategy for medicines control is both important and necessary.

Finding	Response
51. Animal and human diseases are indeed no respecters of administrative boundaries, and the response to them needs to be prompt, well informed and coherent. When we considered all the above issues it seemed to us that they demonstrated some weaknesses in the systems for joint policy-making between London, Cardiff, Edinburgh and Belfast. They also seemed to us to suggest some ways of carrying matters forward. Basic information and analysis need to be shared. Responsibility for disseminating them needs to be clear. Close working between those concerned with animal and human health is highly desirable, and the combined expertise of both senior medical and veterinary staff needs to be drawn on in team building and decision-making. At the same time delays from extended separate consultations have to be avoided. We recognise that the administrative and legislative arrangements covered in this volume have now changed in some significant respects, in particular on animal health and food safety matters, as a consequence of devolution and other events. We would hope that the continuing development of the new relationships and the protocols governing them could take on board the lessons of BSE (Volume 9, paras. 17.42-17.43).	The Government agrees with this recommendation. The creation of the Food Standards Agency has been helpful in this respect. The Government, together with the devolved administrations, will consider whether there is scope for closer working to be achieved.
52. In particular we see merit so far as animal diseases and potential zoonoses are concerned in establishing a clear understanding about: i. the identification of those areas where a uniform and synchronised policy and/or implementation is required and who is to take the lead; ii. the sharing of resources and information; and iii. a structure for consultation and joint decision-making that minimises unnecessary delay (Volume 9, para. 17.44).	The Government is extending the scope of the National Zoonoses Group to cover the devolved administrations (although they previously sent "observers" to meetings).

Finding	Response
53. The sharing of resources and information would assist with the problem we have noted above in the BSE story, that the statutory responsibilities of the Territorial Departments were not well aligned with the resources at their disposal. If there is to be real consensus and not 'follow my leader', information must be more freely available so as to enable the devolved administrations to exercise their responsibilities adequately. We do not suggest that research should be duplicated but rather that the information held by Whitehall should be more routinely and thoroughly disseminated. We note that, since the review of its operation in 1997, SEAC has reported also to Ministers in Wales, Scotland and Northern Ireland. That is certainly to be welcomed (Volume 9, para. 17.46).	Agreed. The Office of Science and Technology's "Guidelines 2000" already emphasise the need for Departments to ensure that they have adequate procedures for early provision and exchange of information on issues which affect more than one Department or agency or have an international dimension.
54. Consistent policy decisions were taken and implemented in relation to BSE largely because the Whitehall CMO and CVO were regarded as having the final word. That final word needed to draw – and indeed did draw – on regular discussions with their colleagues. We believe the quarterly meetings of the CMOs had an especially valuable function as a forum for working through issues of public policy. Ways might be sought of fostering the use of that arrangement in order to assist the provision of consistent, collective advice throughout the UK on animal and human health, recognising that the CMOs may sometimes agree to disagree. Such a forum could also act as a platform for offering collective professional advice direct to other Whitehall Departments (Volume 9, para. 17.49).	The Government agrees that close working between UK CMOs is very important in promoting common understanding of issues in all parts of the country. The Food Standards Agency now has an important role to play in this area.

Finding	Response
55. On a more general point, we believe the BSE story has demonstrated the importance of more open sharing of information and research on all topics. This would not only help to meet public concerns but directly facilitate good policy-making (Volume 9, para. 17.49).	See finding 53.
56. We have considered whether Scotland, like Wales, had other combinations of knowledge and skills to offer that could have assisted UK-wide policy making. It does not appear so. The general approach appears to have been to follow what was suggested in London and to deal with the fall-out. As we have noted on the handling of the SEAC papers, this approach was not fruitful. No arrangement or wish appears to have existed between DAFS and SHHD to consider and interpret the SEAC material with a view to making a proactive contribution to the debate. Dr Kendall's description of totally separate realms of departmental interest on human health on the one hand, and farms and abattoirs on the other, is replicated in the poor liaison arrangements that existed between the two Departments. Within DAFS itself, we were surprised by the avowed lack of knowledge of those dealing with animal health policy, about the meat slaughtering and processing business and about food safety generally. All these are matters which may have been rectified since the period with which we are concerned. We believe it is important that they should have been (Volume 9, para. 11.61).	Devolution has imposed a greater and more direct responsibility on the part of the Scottish Executive to contribute independently to policy-making, and to consider academic and other resources in Scotland that can be utilised as part of the policy-making process. The new Public Health Institute now being established in Scotland will provide a substantial professional resource in the public health area.

The Scottish Executive will also consider whether any further action might be necessary to meet this concern.

The Executive is developing a cross-cutting science strategy, which will be published later this year. |

MEDICINES

Finding	Response
57. Reliance on reported adverse reaction will not result in timely identification of problems arising from disease with long incubation period. A database of concerns other than those resulting from adverse reactions should be considered (Volume 1, para. 1285).	Suspected adverse reaction schemes for human and veterinary medicines are of real and continuing value. MCA is developing a new information management strategy, which will enable the data currently held on different databases to be more accessible and useful in licensing new medicines and monitoring medicines' safety. Consideration will be given as to how data on "concerns" about medicines is gathered and how the information might be shared more widely.
58. The licensing authorities, their advisory committees and others involved in the medicines licensing system each have information and expertise in relation to potential zoonoses that will be of use to the other. Effective action in respect of such diseases depends on this being shared. MAFF, DH and the Medicines Commission should consider what improvements might be needed to existing collaborative arrangements (Volume 1, para. 1285).	Agreed. A number of collaborative arrangements have been developed between MAFF and DH. For example, a National Zoonoses Group has been established to provide an overview and co-ordination of public health action on zoonoses; MAFF chairs an interdepartmental group involving DH, other departments and the devolved administrations, which co-ordinates Government action in relation to risks associated with the use of organophosphates (OPs); and DH chairs a steering group which similarly co-ordinates activity to combat antimicrobial resistance. Both departments have signed a concordat with the Food Standards Agency which ensures that food safety concerns are properly taken into account. The Medicines Commission brings together officials from VMD and MCA. As well as the formal arrangements there are contacts at working level and consideration is already being given to the establishment of a framework to place these contacts on a more formal footing.
59. It is not always clear in practice where responsibility rests as between Ministers, officials and advisory committees for advising, determining policy and taking key decisions on medicines. This should be clarified, so as to ensure that important policy decisions are taken by, or approved by, Ministers, whether those decisions are to take action or to take no action (Volume 1, para. 1285).	In relation to medicines, the law relating to decisions on the authorisation (or withdrawal of authorisation) is clear. The Medicines Commission and other relevant Medicines Act Advisory Bodies (MAAB) offer reasoned advice which is conveyed to Ministers (acting as the Licensing Authority) by officials. Ministers take decisions which are implemented by officials in the Agencies responsible for human (Medicines Control Agency) and veterinary (Veterinary Medicines Directorate) medicinal products. In practice "everyday" regulatory decisions are delegated to the Agencies but it is now routine to refer for decision by Ministers advice which has implications for public or animal health. Practices relating to involving Ministers have been influenced by the experiences of handling the BSE outbreak.
60. The extent of the requirements of confidentiality in relation to the licensing of medicines should be reviewed (Volume 1, para. 1285).	Agreed. The blanket restriction on the release of information stems from Section 118 of the Medicines Act 1968. The Government will consider whether it is appropriate to repeal Section 118 when the Freedom of Information Act 2000 is implemented.

Finding	Response
61. Ring-fencing of medicines decisions to insulate them from outside pressures can reduce accountability. There should be properly reasoned and recorded decision-taking, and the criteria being applied should be made openly available (Volume 1, para. 1285).	Procedures are in place for recording the findings and reasons for advice of the Medicines Act Advisory Bodies (the Medicines Commission, Section 4 Committees and their sub- committees). Medicines' licensing is becoming more open, with the appointment of lay members to the committees and the publication of summary meeting minutes on the Internet, including information on why particular decisions were taken. Obligations to maintain commercial confidentiality and to restrict access to information for operational reasons in advance of a final decision still remain in advance of changes (if any) brought about by implementation of the Freedom of Information Act.
62. Thought should be given to ways of ensuring that those licensing animal derived medicinal products are properly informed about the sources and collection of materials (Volume 1, para. 1285).	For veterinary medicines, guidelines have been in place since 1983 to minimise the risks associated with the potential transmission of pathogens. Data on the source of starting materials of animal origin has been required since the joint CSM and VPC guidelines (applying both to human and veterinary medicines) were introduced in 1989. The European Community guidelines on reducing the risk of transmission of TSEs were given the force of law by way of Commission Directive 1999/104/EEC (for veterinary medicines) and Commission Directive 1999/82/EEC (for human medicines).
63. DTI should review the need to maintain data on products which offer a potential pathway of infection (Volume 1, para. 1286).	The Government agrees with this recommendation. DTI will seek to establish closer links with the Medicines Control Agency to ensure the best possible communications and exchange of information.
64. . . . we had difficulty in pinning down precisely when stocks of products, particularly vaccines, manufactured with UK bovine material were used up. The MCA was not able to provide us with this information and the report of the audit of manufacturers carried out in 1996 did not deal with the issue of phasing out stocks . . . Although there is no evidence at this stage that vaccines or any medicinal products were implicated in transmitting the disease, the possibility cannot be ruled out entirely. Should that be the case, accurate tracing of what happened to products would then be helpful. We found the overall lack of information concerning the phasing out of existing stocks of products frustrating (Volume 7, para. 6.288).	At the time when BSE emerged and prior to the issue of the CSM/VPC guidelines in 1989, industry was not required to keep information on the origin of bovine materials. Records of manufacture are required to be kept for five years after certification (or one year after the expiry of the batch, whichever is longer). Tracing individual batches of vaccines produced in the 1980s to end users would be very difficult and it is hard to identify when batches were exhausted or which patients (or animals) were vaccinated. The Committee on the Safety of Medicines (CSM) will consider the safety of vaccines and BSE-related issues again in the light of the Inquiry's hypothesis that BSE may have emerged in the early 1970s. The CSM's Biologicals Sub-Committee will meet in March to undertake their review. Regulations now in force impose requirements as to record keeping on retailers of veterinary medicinal products intended for food producing animals. Thus, when the review of existing products required by Directive 1999/104/EEC has been completed, there will be a full audit trail from the manufacturer of veterinary medicinal products intended for food producing animals through to the end user.

Finding	Response
65. Even within the blinkers of the false impression on risk, there was undoubtedly room for improvement in the way the guidelines [for industry on BSE and medicines] were followed up. We think it would have been better if . . . There had been clear expectations about reporting to top management and Ministers. We were struck by how little Ministers were informed, let alone consulted, about the massive administrative exercise of following up the guidelines . . . [we were told] that 'Ministers never provided officials with criteria to apply when considering which matters to refer to Ministers. Officials had to apply their own judgement when deciding what matters to refer to Ministers. We believe that Ministers should take a lively interest in what is being done in their name, and that there should be clear presentation to them of important policy decisions (Volume 7, para. 6.368).	See finding 59. Ministers are fully involved in the decision-making process and are consulted on (or participate in) all important decisions. Ministers have also made it clear that they expect decisions with public health implications to be referred to them in a timely manner.
66. Another factor that appears to have left Ministers and senior management in DH in difficulties about accurately tracing and reviewing past actions was defects and gaps in DH record-keeping [on medicines and BSE], ranging from destruction of ministerial papers to the dismal history of its medicines IT system . . . We think it is important that there should be properly reasoned and recorded decision-taking, and that the criteria being applied are made openly available. It should be made plain by whom decisions are actually taken and the basis for these, both on general policy matters and on individual items. And as we have said, important decisions should be validated by Ministers (Volume 7, paras. 6.378-6.379).	See finding 61. Procedures are in place to improve the recording of the findings and reasons for advice given by the Medicines Act Advisory Bodies (the Medicines Commission, Section 4 Committees and their sub- committees).

Finding	Response
67. One of the matters that clearly emerged from the response of the MCA and its committees to BSE was the absence of even rudimentary knowledge about how pharmaceutical materials were obtained from animals, and techniques to ensure they were not contaminated . . . Some of the pharmaceutical manufacturers themselves appear to have been equally uninformed . . . Even less appears to have been known by some of those advising on biological products . . . This was an important knowledge gap among those responding to BSE since the fundamental basis of the UK, and later the European and WHO, approach to both animal and human medicinal products was that clean sources were the only way forward . . . We noted that concerns about its limited knowledge cropped up repeatedly in the BSEWG . . . thought should be given to ensuring that those dealing with medicinal products deriving from animals are informed about the sources and collection of materials (Volume 7, paras. 6.382-6.385).	Agreed. See finding 62. There is work ongoing at EU level too. A proposal for a Directive to regulate manufacturers of starting materials, which has the full support of the UK Government, is currently under discussion.
68. We think that the current variety of different powers over animal health, food safety, medicines and other products should be reviewed to ensure that they offer a means of consistent and prompt action in future when an infected product needs urgently to be removed from circulation (Volume 7, para. 6.390).	See finding 58. The Government believes that appropriate legal powers are already available to protect human and animal health in these circumstances. There is scope for action to be taken quickly and effectively in relation to food, feed, medicines and cosmetics if products are found to be harmful.

Finding	Response

69. Given that it was eventually completed, did the cross-purposes surrounding [the Tyrrell proposals for research into pharmaceuticals] matter . . . we thought that the way the project was handled indicated three lessons for the future: (i). It is important that government itself takes a lead in promoting and disseminating research work needed to determine safety regulatory action. While cooperation with industry may be valuable, it seems to us unrealistic to expect private sector companies to be enthusiastic about promoting and publicising research that could be to their financial detriment. (ii). As we have seen in other fields, there needs to be a clear policy customer for research work . . . When there is more than one customer, and in particular, more than one customer Department, communication between them and the allocation of lead responsibility is essential. (iii). The detachment of the medicines licensing authorities from decision-taking about the Tyrrell studies was striking . . . We think further thought might usefully be given to the arrangements for ensuring their involvement in decision-taking about desirable research on safety matters where animal materials are involved (Volume 7, para. 7.7).

Arrangements are in place to ensure the co-ordination of Government research among departments in cases where issues cross departmental boundaries and/or territorial boundaries. For example, co-ordinating groups on OPs and antimicrobial resistance both have research sub-groups which perform this function.

70. We think that DTI should regularly check that an up-to-date communication system is in place with each of the industries it sponsors to enable it to contact and advise all those who need to know in the event of future questions arising over the safety of an ingredient or process in general use (Volume 7, para. 8.175).

The Government accepts the finding and will consider how this can best be achieved.

Finding	Response
71. We recognise the reasons why so little information exists today in DTI on [relations with the cosmetics industry]. However, it seems to us unfortunate that so little is apparently known about the basic constituents of widely used products of an industry with so many features in common with the pharmaceutical industry. If this information gap still persists, we suggest that it might be reviewed (Volume 7, paras. 8.225-8.227).	The DTI Consumer Affairs Directorate has already improved communication with both the Medicines Control Agency and the Department of Health, and is seeking to ensure that the good relations established will continue. The Department will also review its links with other bodies to see if improvements can be made.

Finding	Response
72. There seemed to us to be several lessons to be drawn from [the consideration of an audit of the uses of cattle tissue] that would apply *pari passu* to other major threats to human and animal health . . . We set out four that struck us particularly in considering the audit:	See finding 73.

- When faced with a deadly cattle disease potentially transmissible to humans, it should have been an immediate priority for MAFF to identify all the ways in which bovine material could come into contact with humans and other animals. This basic information was needed to map the territory that needed to be considered, for risk assessment and for the application of detailed measures. Fact-assembly of this sort ought not to have been confused with research.
- An overview of cattle products needed to transcend Departmental boundaries. Even when the 1996 audit was being put in hand this was heavily orientated to MAFF areas of responsibility. It also needed to draw on a wider range of expertise than that available within Depts alone.
- Overall 'ownership' of exercise needed to be explicit and responsibilities placed on named individuals to direct and follow it through. As part of this, progress reports should not have been regarded as a low-level task to be automatically updated, but treated as a means of accountability. They should have made clear where there were any shortfalls, confusions or failings and who was charged with dealing with them.
- Departmental financial arrangements needed to retain sufficient flexibility to cater for the immediate commissioning of 'soft' research where the need was urgent. This is part of a wider set of issues about the need for modest 'contingency funds' at Departments' discretion for meeting urgent research or consultancy demands (Volume 7, para. 9.189).

NON-FOOD ROUTES OF INFECTION

Finding

Response

73. A comprehensive review to identify all the potential pathways of infection to humans, including those from waste disposal, for a potentially zoonotic disease should be undertaken as a basis for taking steps to prevent transmission. This review should involve all relevant Departments and draw on outside expertise as necessary (Volume 1, para. 1284).

74. An overall handling plan with consistent objectives and a timetable should be drawn up and lead responsibility for dealing with each pathway clearly allocated (Volume 1, para. 1284).

The Environment Agency has already carried out a series of risk assessments on pathways of potentially infected waste material, which were published in June 1997. These included an overview of the risks of BSE via environmental pathways; risks from burning waste MBM from the Over Thirty Months Scheme (OTMS) in power stations; risks from disposing of BSE infected cattle in animal carcass incinerators; an assessment of the risk from BSE carcasses disposed of in landfill sites in the early stages of the epidemic; and an assessment of the risk from waste water disposed of from a rendering plant.

The Government shares the Inquiry's concern and will consider what further action might be necessary. The Environment Agency will review whether there has been a material change in the risk assessment work that has already been done for it, in the light of current knowledge and changing practice, by April 2001.

75. The legislation applicable to different types of product may provide differing and sometimes inconsistent powers for dealing with similar risks or raw materials. Consideration should be given to the need for a power to cut off supply of a widely used but potentially toxic raw material at source (Volume 1, para. 1284).

The Government will review existing specific powers to legislate and take action in response to risks of potentially zoonotic diseases, and will consider whether improvements are necessary.

76. Occupational health risks should be considered in relation to each of those pathways and advice or warnings be promptly provided (Volume 1, para 1284).

Officials from the Ministry of Agriculture, Fisheries and Food, the Department of Health and the Health and Safety Executive will consider developing a Memorandum of Understanding to improve liaison and promote close working as a basis for handling these issues in the future.

77. The HSE should consider means of ensuring that the issue of guidance in respect of risks impacting on different occupations is carried out in a manner which is co-ordinated and expeditious. (Volume 1, para 1287).

The Government accepts this finding. The Health and Safety Executive will undertake a peer review and other activities to consider how guidance can best be developed and issued.

Finding	Response
78. The disposal of waste from any processing of material that may contain the BSE agent should be reviewed to ensure that it does not involve risk of infection of humans or animals (Volume 1, para 1288).	The Government agrees with this finding. MAFF, DETR, the Environment Agency and Water UK will discuss disposal of waste water from rendering plants and commission an independent risk assessment if necessary. Legislation to ban the spreading of untreated waste water from rendering plants is already being prepared and should be in place later this year, following public consultation. Research to investigate wider pathways for disposal of waste from rendering plants and similar processes will be commissioned by DETR and the Environment Agency. The devolved administrations are fully engaged with ongoing activity in this area.
79. [We think the most important lesson for the future] is that identification of pathways along which a transmissible agent might pass should always include waste. This might take many, not all immediately obvious, forms and require diligent tracing through a series of stages. This is likely to require a special exercise carried out on a much wider basis than the sphere of individual Departments (Volume 6, para 10.191).	The Government accepts these findings in principle and will consider what further action needs to be taken. An integrated approach to the assessment of risk posed by a variety of waste disposal routes has already been achieved through the creation of the Environment Agency. Enforcement of various types of environmental controls remains the responsibility of the appropriate authorities, for example, local authorities for air pollution control and water companies for disposal to water. Overall responsibility for ensuring that appropriate waste disposal controls are developed and put in place in England remains with the Department of Environment, Transport and the Regions (DETR), within the legislative framework set by the EU. Equivalent responsibilities have been devolved to Northern Ireland, Scotland and Wales.

See also finding 73. |
| 80. A problem in responding to BSE was the complex and disjointed swathe of arrangements covering land, water and air waste disposal and pollution. Even had a comprehensive overview identified the many waste pathways that needed to be considered, there would have been problems in developing an integrated policy approach. Matters have been improved through the introduction of the Environment Agency. If this has not yet been done, it would be helpful to establish a clear lead role, similar to that exercised by the HSE on occupational risk, for the issue of consistent advice and guidance to those encountering new types of hazardous, or potentially hazardous, animal waste material (Volume 6, para 10.191). | |

Finding	Response

81. It might have been appropriate to consider into which category waste from potentially infective animal tissues might fall. There needs to be a clear mechanism for determining whether particular types of material should be allocated to the 'special' or 'hazardous' waste categories, thus triggering appropriate disposal arrangements. This applies also to cases where, as with BSE, the hazard is potential rather than proven. These are matters on which it would seem wise to clarify general principles and their application in advance of, rather than in the course of, any new threat (Volume 6, para 10.191).

The Government accepts this finding. DETR and the Environment Agency will conduct a consultation exercise on extending the scope of "infectious" (and, therefore, special) waste to cover Group 3, as well as Group 4, biological agents. This could mean that potentially infectious Group 3 wastes will have special requirements imposed if they are likely to spread a disease such as BSE. The consultation exercise will be completed in the next 6-9 months.

82. We found it difficult to distinguish between 'agricultural' and 'controlled' waste in respect of the risks posed by BSE. We were concerned that rendered material spread for agricultural purposes is not apparently a 'controlled waste', as it is in beneficial use, nor is it apparently covered by the provisions concerning rendered SBO material. Suspect tissues and processed materials need consistent consideration and criteria. Where subsequent action differs, it should be on the basis of reasoned analysis (Volume 6, para 10.191).

The Government accepts this finding. There are two relevant EU Directives: the Waste Framework Directive (negotiated by DETR) and the Animal Waste Directive (negotiated by MAFF). Currently, the Animal Waste Directive is being renegotiated to tighten it and at the same time to improve the consistency between it and the Waste Framework Directive. The Directive is due to reach a common position in Summer 2001 and to be implemented by February 2003. Spreading waste on land for agricultural benefit is classified as a waste recovery operation under the Waste Framework Directive. The licensing exemption under which this can be done in practice is currently being reviewed to tighten the controls. The Attorney General has agreed the review of the Court judgement which held that effluent from a rendering plant being spread on agricultural land is not "waste". The UK Agriculture Departments are also bringing forward Regulations to prevent untreated waste water from rendering plants being applied to land. Government and the Environment Agency are giving careful consideration as to which remaining uncertainties need to be evaluated by additional research.

83. We thought that the practice of spreading slaughterhouse and rendering waste on fields, while consistent with notions of recycling, none the less needs review. This would help ensure consistent precautionary procedures and guidance across the UK as a whole against the spread of animal disease or risk to humans (Volume 6, para 10.191).

The Government accepts that this area needs review and has already sought the advice of SEAC. Legislation to ban untreated waste water from rendering plants being applied to land is being prepared. A risk assessment on rendering condensate was commissioned last year. The Government, together with the devolved administrations, will consider what further assessments need to be made and, depending on that, will consider the need for further legislation and controls. Government and the Environment Agency are already carefully considering whether there are other areas which need to be evaluated by additional research.

Finding	Response
84. In the programme of BSE research, work on transmissibility through wastes was notable by its absence. Consistently, with what we have said above, the need for research on this aspect should be given careful consideration, both in relation to BSE and in the event of any future threat of this nature (Volume 6, para 10.191).	The Government accepts this finding. The various regulatory controls applying to the disposal and recovery of waste streams will be reviewed by the Environment Agency, MAFF and DETR to ensure that they work together and are appropriate to current operating practices. See also finding 73.
85. Major changes have taken place in the structure of the waste recycling and disposal system as a result of BSE, in particular the virtual disappearance of knackers for handling fallen stock and the changed nature of the rendering industry. It would be desirable to review the efficacy of the arrangements today and the incentives they provide for the safe disposal of risk material (Volume 6, para 10.191).	The Government shares the Inquiry's concern. Although hunt kennels and knackers still collect fallen stock, the economics of the waste disposal system has already changed significantly as a result of BSE. The Government, together with the devolved administrations, is liaising with representatives of the disposal and farming industries over possible future arrangements for the disposal of fallen stock, although ultimately it is for the livestock industry, like other industries, to work out how best to deal with its waste problems and to pay the associated costs, subject to safety considerations.

The various regulatory controls relating to the disposal and recovery of waste streams will be reviewed by the Environment Agency, MAFF and DETR to ensure that they work together and are appropriate to current operating practices. |
| 86. In considering ways to make the national system of animal disease surveillance and control more effective, as recommended in Volume 2: *Science*, new links between the notification status of disease and associated waste disposal procedures might usefully be explored (Volume 6, para. 10.191). | The Government agrees with this finding. Officials from MAFF, the devolved administrations, DETR and the Environment Agency will consider carcass disposal, the uses of cattle tissues and waste disposal from slaughterhouses and rendering plants as part of the next review of Departmental contingency plans for all notifiable diseases. DETR and the Environment Agency are already looking at the possibility of extending special waste controls to cover Group 3 biological agents. |

RESEARCH

87. Where a problem in animal and human health arises that leads to demands for research of the scale and diversity required by BSE, it is desirable that Government Departments and Agencies coordinate their efforts (Volume 1, para. 1290).

The Government shares the Inquiry's concerns. These are already covered in guidance to departments issued by the Office of Science and Technology: "Guidelines 2000" on scientific advice and policy making. This guidance will also inform the forthcoming Scottish Science Strategy. The TSE Joint Funders Group brings together all the scientists funded by MAFF, DH and the Research Councils to discuss work. The devolved administrations are also part of this process. This allows progress to be kept under review, and serves to identify gaps in the research programme and areas of priority for further funding. The FSA's current review of R&D is helping to address the issue of interdepartmental co-ordination. The Government will consider whether any further guidance might be needed on this point.

88. Coordination of the research effort is desirable in order to achieve: identification of gaps in research; determination of research priorities; identification of the best sources of expert assistance; a well-constructed plan for funding from the outset; competition for research projects; peer review of projects; and efficient arrangements for provision of clinical material researchers (Volume 1, para. 1290).

89. The progress of research and the implications of any new developments must be kept under continuous and open review (Volume 1, para. 1290).

The Government accepts this finding. The Office of Science and Technology's "Guidelines 2000" refers to the need for departments to ask experts to indicate what new information might cause them to review their advice. The point will be taken into account in drawing up the next draft of the Code of Practice for Scientific Advisory Committees.

90. What is now known about the relative sensitivity of mouse bioassay compared with calf bioassay may have implications for the conclusions drawn from mouse bioassays. These need to be reconsidered systematically (Volume 1, para. 1290).

The advice of the Spongiform Encephalopathy Advisory Committee will be sought on this recommendation.

91. Consideration should be given to combining in the same Laboratory research on scientific issues that have common application to human and animal health by scientists practising in each field (Volume 1, para. 1269).

Informal links already exist between those working in government medical and veterinary research establishments. Consideration will be given to whether more formal links may be required.

Finding	Response
92. Our understanding is that the Chief Scientist's 'special fund' could not be used to fund in-house research, and thus could not have been used in this case. However, this episode illustrated to us the tremendous value in having available a small strategic fund that could have been used in such circumstances (Volume 2, para. 7.47).	The Government agrees with the need to move fast to tackle newly identified risks. Some departments have contingency funds under the control of Chief Scientists. Others use different arrangements. All departments believe that existing arrangements are satisfactory once a risk has been identified as sufficiently serious to demand rapid action, but consideration will be given as to any further action needed.
93. An alternative approach would have been to subject the research programme to the overview of an independent research 'supremo' or committee whose remit was, in discussion with MAFF and DH, to coordinate the research and to ensure that contracts were awarded, following open competition, to whoever appeared best able to carry it out appropriately (Volume 2, para. 7.63).	The Government will consider, in conjunction with individual Departments and the Research Councils, what further action might be necessary.
94. An open call for proposals, and strategic overview and coordination of the research, might have been of benefit in this difficult area. A resource centre, charged with the distribution of BSE-affected brain samples, antibodies and other biological reagents might also have been very helpful (Volume 2, para. 7.65).	The Government supports the use of open proposals and competitive tendering. It is looking into how far the "call for proposals" procedure can help in further raising the scientific quality of the research programme in the areas concerned. Through the Joint Funders Group a meeting has been arranged for February 2001. This will presage a new, open call for research proposals on diagnostic development for which the funders have allocated research funding. DH will issue a separate open call later on issues specifically related to public health. A resource centre for reagents has been established at the Institute of Animal Health; the VLA contributes to this. The VLA also has a tissue archive and work is in progress to produce tissues for use in other research, particularly development of diagnostic tests. A similar resource centre for human material is being set up at the NIBSC.

ADVISORY COMMITTEES

<u>Finding</u>

<u>Response</u>

95. An advisory committee should draw a clear distinction between any information provided by others, which it has not reviewed, and its own conclusions (Volume 1, para. 1275).

The Government agrees with this finding. The Office of Science and Technology's "Guidelines 2000" and the proposed Code of Practice for Scientific Advisory Committees both emphasise that experts should explain clearly the reasoning on which their advice is based. The Government will consider whether the next draft of the Code of Practice should be strengthened to ensure that these concerns are further highlighted.

96. An advisory committee should explain the reasoning on which their advice is based (Volume 1, para. 1275).

Since October 1997, the Spongiform Encephalopathy Advisory Committee (SEAC) has published Public Summaries of all its meetings; since November 1998 SEAC has held press conferences with the Chairman and key members around 3 weeks after each meeting. Public Summaries have gradually become more detailed in explaining SEAC's reasoning. Since December 2000, SEAC has published its meeting agendas when the Public Summary is published.

97. When giving advice, an advisory committee should make it clear what principles, if any, of risk management are being applied (Volume 1, para. 1275).

98. An advisory committee should not water down its formulated assessment of risk out of anxiety not to cause public alarm (Volume 1, para. 1275).

The Government agrees with this finding. Any attempt to "water down" an assessment of risk would be incompatible with the principles of openness and transparency at the heart of the Office of Science and Technology's "Guidelines 2000" and underlying the planned Code of Practice for Scientific Advisory Committees.

99. Government Departments must retain 'in house' sufficient scientific expertise to enable them to understand and review advice given by advisory committees (Volume 1, para. 1278).

The Government is carrying out a scoping and exploratory study of 'in house' scientific expertise.

100. Government Departments must review advice given by advisory committees to ensure that the reasons for it are understood and appear to be sound (Volume 1, para. 1278).

The Government agrees with the principle of this finding and will consider whether further guidance to departments is needed on the handling of advice received from advisory committees.

101. Departmental representatives attending meetings of advisory committees in the capacity of secretariat or observers should see that their Departments are promptly informed of any matters which may require a response from government (Volume 1, para. 1279).

The Government accepts this finding and will look to reflect it in finalising the Code of Practice for Scientific Advisory Committees.

Finding	Response
102. Contingency planning is a vital part of government. The existence of advisory committees is not an alternative to this. The advisory committees should, where their advice will be of value, be asked to assist in contingency planning (Volume 1, para. 1279).	The Government recognises the importance of effective contingency planning – departments have a responsibility to ensure an appropriate level of preparedness. The Government will consider what further action might be necessary to clarify how advisory committees may assist in the planning process. For example, SEAC is already involved in sheep contingency planning and has expressed a wish to be more pro-active in identifying future problems that should be brought to the attention of Government departments and devolved administrations.
103. Advisory committees set up to advise on problems of animal health, or animal and human health, which are common throughout the United Kingdom should report to the appropriate Departments both in England and in the Territories (Volume 1, para. 1282).	This is done already in most cases. The Government will consider, in consultation with the devolved administrations, whether further action or advice is necessary.
104. The areas of advice that are required from the advisory committee should be identified as precisely as possible before the committee is set up (Volume 1, para. 1291). 105. The terms of reference should specify with as much precision as possible the role of the committee (Volume 1, para. 1291).	These points are already addressed in the Office of Science and Technology's "Guidelines 2000". The Government will consider how best to reflect and clarify them in the second draft of the Code of Practice for Scientific Advisory Committees. The Government will review SEAC's terms of reference, especially in relation to giving advice to the public.
106. The composition of the committee should include experts in the areas of the advice that is likely to be required (Volume 1, para. 1291).	This point is already addressed in general terms in the Office of Science and Technology's "Guidelines 2000" and will be reflected more specifically in the next draft of the Code of Practice for Scientific Advisory Committees.
107. Those invited to join a committee should be given a realistic estimate of the commitment required (Volume 1, para. 1291).	The Government accepts this recommendation in principle and will consider whether further guidance to departments is necessary.
108. Government should seek advice from the professional or other body best qualified to advise on suitable candidates for membership (Volume 1, para. 1291).	The general principles on the identification of appropriate experts are already covered in the OST's "Guidelines 2000", which suggest that departments should consult, among others, learned societies and professional bodies so as to draw on a sufficiently wide range of experts. The Government will consider placing this on a more formal basis.

Finding	Response
109. Potential conflicts of interest should not preclude selection of those members otherwise best qualified, but conflicts of interest should be declared and registered (Volume 1, para. 1291).	The Government's current policy mirrors this approach. It is set out in Guidance on Codes of Practice for Board Members of Public Bodies. In addition the Commissioner for Public Appointments' Guidance requires possible conflicts of interest to be explored fully at the time of recruitment. The Government reviews this policy from time to time and has also consulted on this issue in preparing the Code of Practice for Scientific Advisory Committees.
110. Where any item of business involves an apparent conflict of interest on the part of a member, that should be declared (Volume 1, para. 1291).	
111. Where the workload of a committee is considerable, it is reasonable that members who are not public servants should be remunerated (Volume 1, para. 1291).	The Government accepts this finding in principle and will consider further how it can best be achieved. In some cases, committee members do receive remuneration for their efforts as well as expenses.
112. It will often be desirable to draw the secretariat from the commissioning Department(s) in order to provide a two-way channel of communication (Volume 1, para. 1291).	The Government agrees with these findings. This is already common practice in most cases, but the Government will ensure that the Inquiry's concerns are specifically taken into account when issuing the next draft of the Code of Practice for Scientific Advisory Committees.
113. In such cases, as in all cases, the secretariat must be careful to respect the independence of the committee (Volume 1, para. 1291).	
114. Where a policy decision is urgent, consideration should be given to whether delaying the decision pending advice from an advisory committee is the best course (Volume 1, para. 1291).	The Government accepts the need to act quickly when an issue is urgent, but believes that, in practice, expert advice can be assembled rapidly on an *ad hoc* basis where there is an urgent need to do so. While such advice may not be as comprehensive as that of a properly constituted committee, it is likely to be better than relying on in-house expertise alone, and can be reviewed at a later date.
115. Consideration should be given at the outset to the manner in which the committee will contribute to deciding policy (Volume 1, para. 1291).	The Government accepts this finding in principle. The general concern is already addressed in the Office of Science and Technology's "Guidelines 2000". The Government will consider whether the next draft of the Code of Practice for Scientific Advisory Committees needs to be more specific on this point.

Finding	Response
116. Government should recognise that if a committee is asked to advise which policy option to adopt, there may be little alternative but to follow the advice given (Volume 1, para. 1291).	The Government notes this comment.
117. Where the policy decision involves the balancing of considerations which fall outside the expertise of the committee, it will normally not be appropriate to ask the committee to advise which policy option to adopt (Volume 1, para. 1291).	The Government accepts these findings. The Office of Science and Technology's "Guidelines 2000" emphasises, for example, the need for the limits of an expert's responsibilities for advice to be made clear. The point is being taken into account in the drafts of the Code of Practice for Scientific Advisory Committees.
118. It may be appropriate to set out a range of policy options, together with the implications of each (Volume 1, para. 1291).	
119. Where advice is sought on the implications of policy options, this may best be achieved by dialogue between government and the committee (Volume 1, para. 1291)	The Government agrees with this finding and will seek to address it in the next draft of the Code of Practice for Scientific Advisory Committees.
120. Where advice is required only on those ingredients of a policy decision which fall within the particular expertise of the committee, questions should be formulated with precision to achieve that result (Volume 1, para. 1291).	The Government accepts this finding, which is already covered in general terms in the "Guidelines 2000" and the July 2000 Report of Sir Robert May's Review of Risk Procedures Used by the Government's Advisory Committees Dealing with Food Safety. The point will also be reflected in the next draft of the Code of Practice for Scientific Advisory Committees.
121. Where a Department has concerns about the practical implications of advice that a committee may give, these should be placed openly before the committee (Volume 1, para. 1291).	The Government accepts this finding in principle and will consider what further action might be necessary.
122. Where a committee is asked to advise on risk management, it will normally be helpful for the committee to follow a formal structure based on recognised principles of risk assessment (Volume 1, para. 1291).	The Government accepts this finding and will seek to take it into account in the next draft of the Code of Practice for Scientific Advisory Committees.

Finding	Response
123. Advice should normally be given in writing (Volume 1, para. 1291).	The Government accepts this finding in principle and will seek to cover it in the next draft of the Code of Practice for Scientific Advisory Committees. Account will need to be taken of situations where urgent advice may be required.
124. Advice should be in terms that can be understood by a layperson (Volume 1, para. 1291).	The Government accepts this finding in principle and will seek to cover it in the next draft of the Code of Practice for Scientific Advisory Committees.
125. Advice should clearly state the reasons for conclusions (Volume 1, para. 1291).	This is covered already in the Office of Science and Technology's "Guidelines 2000". It will also be addressed when preparing the next draft of the Code of Practice for Scientific Advisory Committees.
126. Assumptions underlying advice should be made clear (Volume 1, para. 1291).	The Government accepts this finding and will ensure that it is covered in the next draft of the Code of Practice for Scientific Advisory Committees.
127. Advice should identify the nature and extent of any areas of uncertainty (Volume 1, para. 1291). 128. Where appropriate, the advice should set out the different policy options and the implications of each (Volume 1, para. 1291).	These points are already covered in the Office of Science and Technology's "Guidelines 2000" and are being reflected in the drafts of the Code of Practice for Scientific Advisory Committees.
129. The advice of the committee, together with any papers necessary for the full understanding of that advice, should be circulated to all within government with responsibility for policy decisions in respect of which the advice is relevant (Volume 1, para. 1291).	Papers are routinely circulated around interested Government departments, including the devolved administrations. The Government will consider whether there is a need for any supplementary guidance on the internal handling of scientific advice by departments, once received.
130. The advice of the committee should normally be made public by the committee (Volume 1, para. 1291).	The Government accepts this recommendation. This is done already in most cases, but the Government will seek to ensure that the point is specifically covered in the next draft of the Code of Practice for Scientific Advisory Committees. The Freedom of Information Act 2000 is also relevant here.
131. The proceedings of the committee should be as open as is compatible with the requirements of confidentiality (Volume 1, para. 1291).	This is already is covered in the draft Code of Practice for Scientific Advisory Committees. Since 1997 the Government has firmly encouraged the opening up of scientific advisory committees and a lot of scientific advice to government is put into the public domain.

Finding	Response
132. Departments should retain 'in house' sufficient expertise to ensure that the advice of advisory committees, and the reasoning behind it, can be understood and evaluated (Volume 1, para. 1291).	See comment for finding 99.
133. Advice given by a committee should be reviewed by those to whom it is given to ensure that the reasons for the advice are understood and appear sound (Volume 1, para. 1291).	See comments for findings 100 and 129.
134. Where the reasoning of the advice of a committee is unclear, clarification should be obtained from the committee (Volume 1, para. 1291).	See comments for findings 100, 118 and 133.
135. The advice and reasoning of advisory committees should be made public (Volume 1, para. 1302).	The Government will ensure this point is covered, as necessary, in the next draft of the Code of Practice for Scientific Advisory Committees. The Freedom of Information Act 2000 will also be relevant here.
136. Any advice given by a CMO or advisory committee should be, and be seen to be, objective and independent of government (Volume 1, para. 1302).	The Government agrees. Insofar as it relates to committees, the point will be reflected in the draft Code of Practice for Scientific Advisory Committees.
137. Our examination of both formal and informal advice given by SEAC suggests a need to identify, either generally or on specific issues, all those within government with responsibility for policy decisions to which the advice is relevant. They can then be sent relevant minutes and more formal 'advices', and any papers necessary to understand them (Volume 11, para. 4.766).	The Government accepts this finding in principle. Consideration will be given as to how this can best be implemented.
138. Witnesses representing consumer interests made the point that a lay member can play a vital role on an expert committee, and in particular can ensure that advice given by the committee addresses the concerns of, and is in a form that is intelligible to, the public. There is force in this (Volume 11, para. 4.773).	The Government agrees with this finding. Lay members have already been appointed to many of the Government's scientific advisory committees. The issue is covered in the Office of Science and Technology's "Guidelines 2000" and will be taken into account in the next draft of the Code of Practice for Scientific Advisory Committees.

RISK MANAGEMENT AND COMMUNICATION

Finding	Response
139. Reliance on a trade association or other body to communicate the importance of a precautionary measure is not always appropriate (Volume 1, para. 1273).	The Government agrees with this finding. For food safety measures, multiple routes of communication are normally used. Farming unions, manufacturing and/or retail trade organisations are a very quick and effective means of getting messages out and between them cover a very significant fraction of all food businesses. Communication through Local Authority enforcers, in parallel, provides an alternative route to individual small businesses. Openness and good communications with the media also help to ensure that the right messages are promulgated widely.
140. The trust that the public has in the Chief Medical Officers is precious and should not be put at risk (Volume 1, para. 1301).	The Government agrees with this finding.
141. The role, if any, of the Chief Veterinary Officer in making public statements in relation to risk to human health from a zoonosis or potential zoonosis should be clarified (Volume 1, para. 1301).	In relation to zoonoses, the CVO's responsibility is to provide advice, information and policy input on the disease situation in animals and to advise on the extent to which animals or their products may pose a risk to the public. The CVO is therefore responsible for identifying hazards and contributing to risk assessment. The CVO is able to engage in direct communication with the public, giving advice and information on veterinary matters and the control of animal diseases.
142. BSE is a novel and alarming zoonosis. There is much about it that is not yet understood. Precautionary measures need to be applied to reduce the potential risk as low as is reasonably practicable (Volume 1, para. 1264).	The Food Standards Agency has recently completed a full review of controls on BSE with a view to ensuring that all necessary measures for protecting human and animal health are in place.
143. Although likelihood of a risk to human life may appear remote, where there is uncertainty all reasonably practicable precautions should be taken (Volume 1, para. 1283). 144. Precautionary measures should be strictly enforced even if the risk that they address appears to be remote (Volume 1, para. 1283).	The Government is committed to applying the precautionary principle where appropriate. Measures to improve communication with enforcers and to monitor effectiveness of enforcement are already in place in the food safety area via the Food Standards Agency.

Finding	Response
145. Where policy decisions turn on risks to human health, DH should be involved in the formulation of policy from the outset (Volume 1, para. 1274).	The Government accepts this finding. Good relationships already exist between UK Agriculture and Health Departments. Consideration will be given to placing these on a more formal basis. Furthermore, departments are applying Health Impact Assessments whenever their policies are likely to affect human health.
146. Reference to outside expert committees involves delay. It should be avoided, where possible, in a situation of urgency (Volume 1, para. 1274).	The Government agrees that it is essential to move quickly to take expert advice on an *ad hoc* basis where there is an urgent need to do so. This is in addition to the "in-house" expertise within departments.
147. When a precautionary measure is introduced, rigorous thought must be given to every aspect of its operation with a view to ensuring that it is watertight and fully effective (Volume 1, para. 1273).	See comments for finding 144.
148. If this cannot be done before the measure is introduced, it should be done as soon as possible afterwards (Volume 1, para. 1276).	
149. To establish credibility it is necessary to generate trust (Volume 1, para. 1302).	The Government accepts these findings. Over time there has been a significant loss of public confidence in the way that government handled food safety. The creation of the Food Standards Agency is a major step towards restoring public trust. The Agency's statutory powers, e.g. to publish its advice, demonstrate the Government's commitment to openness in this area. The Agency has established working practices of openness and honesty, and of consulting widely before making decisions, to help re-establish public trust, e.g. holding Board meetings in public, reviewing of BSE controls in a fully public way; the FSA Code of Practice on Openness provides useful information on the Agency's approach.
150. Trust can only be generated by openness (Volume 1, para. 1302).	
	In relation to science, the importance of openness and trust is also stressed throughout the Office of Science and Technology's "Guidelines 2000".
151. Openness requires recognition of uncertainty, where it exists (Volume 1, para. 1302).	The Government shares the Inquiry's concern. This point is emphasised in the Office of Science and Technology's "Guidelines 2000". The Government is operating on the basis of the need to be open about scientific uncertainty and is exploring better ways of communicating this to the public.
152. The importance of precautionary measures should not be played down on the grounds that the risk is unproved (Volume 1, para. 1302).	The Government accepts this finding. Precautionary measures may be taken when there is uncertainty and the level of risk is unknown or unproven. As indicated above, it is fully accepted that steps must be taken to ensure that precautionary measures are implemented effectively. The Food Standards Agency will be looking further at the ways in which advice in a situation of uncertainty can best be obtained as part of a review of expert advice planned for later this year.

Finding	Response
153. The public should be trusted to respond rationally to openness (Volume 1, para. 1302).	Agreed. The Government has made it a priority to encourage a culture of openness, trusting the public and stimulating informed public debate; for example, by establishing the independent Food Standards Agency and opening up scientific advisory committees, including the appointment of consumer representatives. A great deal of scientific advice to Government is put into the public domain. The Freedom of Information Act 2000 is also relevant here.
154. Scientific investigation of risk should be open and transparent (Volume 1, para. 1302).	Agreed. The need for transparency and to publish evidence on which a decision is based are principles which run throughout the Office of Science and Technology's "Guidelines 2000" on scientific advice and policy making. They are also covered in the Code of Practice for Scientific Advisory Committee and the July 2000 report of Sir Robert May's group on the "Review of Risk Procedures Used by the Government's Advisory Committees Dealing with Food Safety." It also fits with the approach to risk communication advocated by the Interdepartmental Liaison Group on Risk Assessment (ILGRA) and the Department of Health.
155. Where a precautionary measure is introduced, rigorous thought must be given to every aspect of its operation with a view to ensuring that it is fully effective and its purpose and application understood by those concerned (Volume 1, para. 1273).	Agreed. Once a decision is taken to introduce any measure to protect public health, consultation with all stakeholders (including both enforcers and those affected) should be undertaken to ensure that all relevant factors are taken into account to ensure full effectiveness. Openness and good communication are important and necessary to ensure that the purpose of the measures and their application are properly understood by all concerned.

LEGISLATION

156. Where an animal disease is identified, which could be transmitted to animals or humans via a range of possible routes, powers under UK and European law which enable Ministers to order the slaughter of animals, and the destruction of animal tissues or anything which might carry infection, should not be restricted merely because it cannot be established as a reasonable probability, as opposed to a mere possibility: that the disease is transmissible; or that a particular animal may be infected by the disease in question; or that particular organs or tissues in an animal may carry infection (Volume 1, para. 1329).

157. Similarly, any powers under UK and European law which enable Ministers to adopt an alternative approach of banning the use of any substances for particular purposes in order to protect human or animal health should not be restricted merely because one or more of the matters referred to above cannot be established as a reasonable probability, as opposed to a mere possibility (Volume 1, para. 1329).

The Government believes that in all reasonably foreseeable circumstances it will have the legal powers to act proportionately to take protective measures in response to new hazards, even where they are uncertain.

158. Medicines and consumer legislation should be reviewed so Government has the power to act swiftly and comprehensively to ban substances or processes posing risk to human health (Volume 1, para. 1329).

The Government shares the Inquiry's concern. Existing legislation already provides effective powers to act swiftly and comprehensively to ban substances or processes posing a risk to human health. In the medicines field, under existing EU legislation both human and veterinary medicines can be quickly removed from the market by revoking or suspending the relevant marketing authorisation (licence). This can be done immediately if there is a serious danger to health. The Government will consider whether any further action needs to be taken in relation to consumer legislation.

Finding	Response
159. Government should review and clarify its powers under European law to introduce emergency measures for the protection of animal and public health in relation to outbreaks of disease where measures have previously been taken by the European Commission (Volume 1, para. 1329).	The Government does not believe there are any serious gaps in its powers to take proportionate emergency action against hazards to human or animal health in relation to animals and animal products and food. The existing harmonised Community rules which safeguard public and animal health at Community level already permit appropriate national controls in respect of new outbreaks or where new hazards arise which were not contemplated by existing Community measures.
160. A point of law was raised in relation to the SBO (Amendment) Order 1995. Once definitive measures for a relevant outbreak of disease were adopted by the European Commission at the community level, it followed that Member States were no longer entitled to adopt unilateral measures. This point sufficiently impressed the judge to lead to grant of leave to seek Judicial Review. The possibility that urgent measures of this kind should be open to challenge on the grounds that they were impermissible under European law is a matter of concern (Volume 6, para. 7.203).	
161. If there remains any danger that emergency measures may be readily susceptible to challenge by way of judicial review in this way, we think it desirable to consider steps which might minimise this danger (Volume 6, para. 7.203).	

VARIANT CJD

162. The needs of victims of vCJD and their families have special features. Consideration should be given to how best the health and welfare services can meet them. Patients for whom a care plan has been carefully have received better management than those for whom this is lacking. What is needed includes:

- as speedy as possible a diagnosis of vCJD;
- informed and sympathetic advice to relatives about the future course of the disease and the needs of the patient;
- speedy assistance for those who wish to care for the victim at home. Needs often include aids for the care of the disabled, modification to the home, financial assistance and respite care;
- a coordinated care package which addresses the needs of the victims and their families; and, if requested
- a suitable institutional environment for a young person, incapacitated and terminally ill. (Volume 1, paras. 1283, 1338).

See comments for finding 167.

163. All pathways by which vCJD may be transmitted between humans must be identified and all reasonably practicable measures taken to block them (Volume 1, para. 1283).

The Government shares the Inquiry's concern. Measures have already been taken, on the basis of expert advice, to reduce the theoretical risk of vCJD transmission via blood and blood products. The Department of Health is agreeing action plans on decontamination with individual NHS Trusts to ensure that they meet agreed standards. Similar action is in train in the devolved administrations. Single-use surgical instruments for tonsillectomies will be phased in during 2001. Consideration will be given to any further action needed to reduce risks; for example, sourcing of clinical Fresh Frozen Plasma in relation to vCJD transmission via blood.

Finding	Response

164. Batches of vaccines manufactured during the 1970s cannot . . . be ruled out as a source of infection merely because of their date of manufacture. Patients with vCJD born before 1960 are unlikely to have been infected by childhood vaccination, but the possibility of infection via vaccinations in adulthood may merit consideration . . . These possibilities should be taken into account in an analysis of the specific batches of vaccines administered to victims of vCJD, and consideration given to whether there is any common batch or other factor (Volume 8, para. 5.185).

This is done already. The national CJD Surveillance Unit routinely investigates the full medical history of all patients, including medical injections. So far, no links have been found.

165. An *ad hoc* Working Party of the Committee on Safety of Medicines . . . noted that both human and cattle vaccines prepared with UK-sourced bovine materials have been widely distributed throughout Western Europe without apparently being associated with outbreaks of either vCJD or BSE. This is taken as a strong argument against the possibility that vaccines have been vectors of either disease . . . It will be apparent that some of the assumptions made by the Working Party of the CSM are open to question for reasons we have set out in our Report. We hope that government will look at the topic again in the light of our comments (Volume 8, paras. 5.186-5.187).

The Government shares the Inquiry's concern. In March 2000, Ministers asked the Committee on the Safety of Medicines to investigate the safety of vaccines prepared with UK-sourced bovine materials from 1980 onwards on the (worst case) assumption that vaccines might be a possible vector of BSE or vCJD. The Government has asked the Committee on the Safety of Medicines (CSM) to consider the safety of vaccines and BSE-related issues in the light of the Inquiry's hypothesis that BSE might have emerged in the early 1970s. The Biologicals Sub-Committee of the CSM will meet in March 2001 to undertake their review.

Finding	Response
166. The 1999 Annual report of CJDSU draws attention to the geographical distribution of cases of vCJD (see Figure 5.1, in which the data have been further updated) and shows that if the UK is divided into 'North' and 'South' regions, the rate per million individuals aged between 16 and 54, is 2.57 for the 'North' region and 1.30 per million individuals for the 'South'. . . We hope that the opportunity to investigate such clusters will provide information on common factors and lead to a firm conclusion about the source of infection and its route to affected patients. Such knowledge will improve understanding of the disease and hopefully lead to strategies for treatment (Volume 8, para. 5.188).	A protocol has been developed for identifying possible linked cases and investigating at local and national levels to see whether there are potential implications in relation to the way that vCJD is spread. An investigation of 5 potentially linked cases in Leicestershire is due to report this spring. Experience gained will be invaluable for any similar investigations in the future.

167. It seems that patients for whom a care plan had been carefully arranged have received better management than those for whom this was lacking. It should be possible for all suspected vCJD cases to receive such a care plan now that a care co-ordinator has been appointed by the CJDSU to provide advice to statutory care providers in both the health and social services sectors and to act as an advocate on behalf of patients with vCJD and their families (Volume 8, para. 6.205).

The Government have established a new national fund for the care of victims of vCJD. The fund will ensure a speedy response following diagnosis and improvements in the quality of care for patients. The new care package is not intended to replace local services but to supplement gaps in local service provision. The intention is to support patients in the community, using the fund to pay for those elements of the care package that cannot be readily supplied by local health and social services. A care co-ordinator from the CJD Surveillance Unit will be asked to look at each patient's package of care following attendance at a case conference arranged by a Key Worker. They will agree the care package and make a decision on whether additional money is needed from the central pot to make good any local deficiencies. In addition, Health Departments are:

–   establishing a 'virtual' network of knowledgeable and experienced individuals who can be called upon to provide information and advice;

–   enhancing staff levels with the CJDSU;

–   preparing guidance for the NHS and Social Services;

–   ensuring close working with the voluntary organisations and families of CJD patients to make certain that the care package is effective and properly meets people's needs.

PUBLIC HEALTH MEASURES – BSE & vCJD

This annex sets out in summary the measures in place to protect the public.

BSE: Public Health Measures

- cattle suspected of having BSE are compulsorily slaughtered and their carcasses are destroyed;

- milk produced by cows which are suspected of having BSE may not be used for human consumption;

- controls on Specified Risk Material (SRM) prohibit the use of certain specified animal products which are known to, or might theoretically, harbour BSE infectivity;

- SRM controls are in place for imported beef, sheep meat, goat meat and certain other products of animal origin;

- vertebral columns from cattle, sheep and goats cannot be used to make products for human consumption. In particular this includes mechanically recovered meat;

- meat from cattle over thirty months old at slaughter may not be sold for human consumption (with certain specified exceptions); and

- beef bones from cattle over six months old, which originated in this country, may not be used in the manufacture of food or food products which are not supplied direct to the ultimate consumer.

Medicines and Vaccines:

- guidelines control the use of bovine materials in the manufacture of human and veterinary medicines, including vaccines. These will shortly have the force of law – from 1 March 2001 for human medicines, and from 1 June 2001 for veterinary medicines;

- the Medicines Control Agency and the Veterinary Medicines Directorate have asked all manufacturers of licensed medicinal products (human and veterinary) to confirm that all their products comply with the latest guidelines; and,

- the Government has asked for a comprehensive assessment of vaccine safety and bovine material.

Variant CJD: reducing theoretical risk of transmission between humans

Measures already in progress:

- leucodepletion of all blood for transfusion;

- use of imported plasma to manufacture blood products;

- single-use instruments for tonsillectomy; and,

- decontamination action plan for all NHS Trusts.

Measures under consideration:

- sourcing of clinical fresh frozen plasma.

Animal Health Measures

- mammalian protein (with specific exceptions) is prohibited in any ruminant feed;

- MMBM is prohibited in any farmed livestock feed;

- MMBM material is banned, except in tightly defined circumstances, on premises where livestock feed is used, produced or stored;

- those handling MMBM material are required thoroughly to clean and disinfect their premises/equipment and keep comprehensive records;

- the feed ban is monitored by extensive surveillance carried out by the State Veterinary Service and the DARD Veterinary Service;

- SRM may not be fed to any creature;

- MMBM may not be incorporated in fertiliser for agricultural use;

- offspring of BSE confirmed cases are traced and destroyed;

- cattle suspected of having BSE are compulsorily slaughtered and their carcasses are destroyed;

- milk produced by cows which are suspected of having BSE may not be used for any purpose other than feeding the cow's own calf.

STRATEGIC SCIENCE POLICY CO-ORDINATION

1.   The Government has established structures to enable it to take a strategic overview of the framework in which research is commissioned, and scientific advice is handled. These are regularly reviewed through the publication of the Forward Look of government-funded science, engineering and technology and the reports on the implementation of Guidelines on the use of Scientific Advice in Policy Making (now Guidelines 2000).

2.   The Government's Chief Scientific Adviser (CSA) is responsible to the Prime Minister and members of the Cabinet for the quality of scientific advice within Government and for providing personal advice to them on any aspect of the Government's policy on science and technology. The Chief Medical Officer is the chief medical adviser to the UK Government. In particular, the CSA has responsibility for the Government's guidelines on advice and policy making on science and technology and for their implementation; for ensuring the co-ordination of science policy issues within Government and with the devolved administrations; for maintaining an overview of Government policies affecting the UK science base; and for the Government's international science and technology policy including co-ordinating the UK's position on EU framework programmes.

3.   The Chief Scientific Adviser's Committee (CSAC) is a regular forum for departmental chief scientists and senior officials with responsibility for R&D, under the chairmanship of the CSA. Its remit is to consider issues of relevance to the Government and the devolved administrations concerning science, engineering and technology (SE&T). In particular:

  •   To provide advice to Ministers, primarily through the Ministerial Science Group.

  •   To discuss and facilitate implementation of policy on SE&T.

  •   To identify and promulgate good practice in SE&T-related areas, including the use of scientific advice in policy making.

  •   To facilitate communication on particular high profile SE&T-related issues and those posing new challenges for Government.

4.   The Ministerial Science Group (MSG), chaired by the Minister for Science and Innovation, comprises Ministers from each of the departments with significant SET activity, including the devolved administrations. It aims to promote a co-ordinated and coherent approach to SET policy-making. The Office of Science and Technology (OST) provides the secretariat. Where issues cross departmental boundaries, responsibility for high-level co-ordination of the policy on particular issues may rest with the appropriate Ministerial committee. This may be one of the standing Cabinet Committees such as HS or EA or a specially convened committee such as MISC6 – the Ministerial Group on Biotechnology and Genetic

Modification whose role is to consider issues relating to biotechnology, in particular those arising from genetic modification.

5. The Council for Science and Technology (CST) acts as the Prime Minister's top level advisory body on the strategic policies and framework for science and technology in the UK and on medium to longer term strategic science and technology issues.

Research Management and Co-ordination

6. Each department is responsible for commissioning research to inform and support policy formulation and evaluation and regulatory activities. They fund research according to their overall policy and research priorities from within their budgets. Research may be commissioned in-house, in a government-owned laboratory, or externally through universities, Research Council institutes or other independent contractors.

7. Where an issue covers the interests of more than one department, the departments concerned retain primary responsibility for commissioning the research they need for their specific policy and regulatory functions, but they should co-ordinate their efforts. Where one department has a clear policy lead, it will normally lead on research co-ordination. For example, DH leads on the research funders group on TSEs and DETR leads on the issue of global environmental change.

8. The co-ordination of research between government bodies may also be governed by formal arrangements. For example, some departments have high-level agreements with the devolved administrations which cover research co-ordination. Departments may also have concordats with other government departments and with the research councils for the same purpose.

9. For particular issues research co-ordination is handled by co-ordinating committees. For research into TSEs the responsible committee is the High Level Committee to Monitor the Progress on Research Relating to TSEs chaired by the Cabinet Secretary. This is supported by the TSEs R&D Funders Group chaired by the Director of R&D from the Department of Health.

10. The CSA may call departments and Research Councils together to ensure that proper arrangements for co-ordination are in hand, particularly where there is no clear lead.

11. Increasingly decisions on policy and regulation are made at the EU level. Government departments are generally responsible for ensuring that the UK position is properly represented in the EU institutions and this effort is co-ordinated by the European Secretariat of the Cabinet Office.

REFERENCES AND USEFUL PUBLICATIONS

- *Report of the BSE Inquiry*, Stationery Office, October 2000
  (http://www.bseinquiry.gov.uk)

- *Modernising Government White Paper*, Cabinet Office, March 1999

- *First Report of the Committee on Standards In Public Life*, HMSO, 1996

- *The Commissioner for Public Appointments' Guidance on Appointments to Public Bodies*, Office of the Commissioner for Public Appointments, July 1998

- *Guidance on Codes of Practice for Board Members of Public Bodies,* Cabinet Office, February 2000

- *The Civil Service Code*, Cabinet Office

- *Guidelines for UK Government Websites*, Cabinet Office, December 1999

- *How to Conduct Written Consultation Exercises: An Introduction for Central Government*, Cabinet Office, April 2000

- *Guidelines 2000: Scientific Advice and Policy Making*, Office of Science and Technology, July 2000
  (http://www.dti.gov.uk/ost)

- *A Consultation Document on a Code of Practice for Scientific Advisory Committees*, Office of Science and Technology, July 2000
  (http://www.dti.gov.uk/ost)

- *Review of Science and Technology Activity Across Government*, Council for Science and Technology, July 1999

- *Government Implementation Plan In Response to the Council for Science and Technology Report: Review of Science and Technology Activity Across Government*, Office of Science and Technology, July 2000

- *Science and Innovation White Paper: Excellence and Opportunity: A Science and Innovation Policy for the 21st Century*, Office of Science and Technology, July 2000

- *Review of Risk Procedures Used by the Government's Advisory Committees Dealing with Food Safety*, Office of Science and Technology, July 2000
  (http://www.dti.gov.uk/ost)

- *Risk Assessment and Risk Management: Improving Policy and Practice Within Government Departments*, ILGRA, HSE Books, December 1998
  (http://www.hse.gov.uk/dst/ilgra.htm)

- *Risk Communication: A Guide to Regulatory Practice*, ILGRA, 1998
  (http://www.hse.gov.uk/dst/ilgra.htm)

- *Communicating About Risks to Public Health: Pointers to Good Practice*, Stationery
  Office, 1998

- *Management of Risk – A Strategic Overview,* HM Treasury, January 2001

- *BSE in Great Britain: A Progress Report*, MAFF, June 2000
  (http://www.maff.gov.uk/animalh/bse)

- *Strategy For Research and Development Relating to the Animal Health Aspects of
  Transmissible Spongiform Encephalopathies*, MAFF/DH, July 1998
  (http://www.maff.gov.uk/animalh/bse)

- *The Food Standards Act 1999*, HMSO, 1999
  (http://www.legislation.hmso.gov.uk/acts/acts19990028.htm)

- *The Food Standards Act: Explanatory Notes*, HMSO, 1999
  (http://www.legislation.hmso.gov.uk/acts/en/1999en28.htm)

- *Food Standards Agency Review of BSE Controls*, December 2000
  (http://www.bsereview.org.uk)

- *Freedom of Information Act 2000*, HMSO
  (http://www.hmso.gov.uk)

GLOSSARY

Many of the definitions in this glossary are quoted directly from the BSE Inquiry Report (Volume 16, "Reference Material").

Term or abbreviation	Meaning
ACDP	Advisory Committee on Dangerous Pathogens, established in 1981 to advise the Health and Safety Executive on all aspects of hazards and risks to workers and others from exposure to pathogens.
Attack rate	The number of animals in an experimental group which succumb to a disease after exposure of the group to an infectious agent.
BBSRC	Biotechnology and Biological Sciences Research Council, established in April 1994.
BSE	Bovine Spongiform Encephalopathy, a slowly progressive and ultimately fatal neurological disorder of adult cattle.
CDSC	Communicable Disease Surveillance Centre. Responsible for monitoring human infectious diseases.
CJD	Creutzfeld-Jakob Disease, a human transmissible spongiform encephalopathy.
CJD Surveillance Unit (CJDSU)	Research Unit set up in Edinburgh in 1990. It administers a national surveillance programme for CJD in the UK and acts as an information resource for carers and professionals.
CMO	Chief Medical Officer.
CSA	Chief Scientific Adviser. Head of the Office of Science and Technology.
CSAC	Chief Scientific Adviser's Committee. Considers issues of relevance to the Government and the devolved administrations concerning science, engineering and technology.

CST	Council for Science and Technology. Advises Government on the strategic policies and framework for science and technology in the UK.
CVL	Central Veterinary Laboratory. Now part of the VLA. Responsible for co-ordinating the surveillance and investigation of animal diseases.
CVO	Chief Veterinary Officer.
DARD	Department of Agriculture and Rural Development in Northern Ireland.
DETR	Department of the Environment, Transport and the Regions.
DH, DoH	Department of Health.
DTI	Department of Trade and Industry.
EA	Environment Agency (for England and Wales).
Epidemiology	The statistical study of categories of persons or animals and the patterns of disease from which they suffer, with the aim of determining the events or circumstances causing those diseases.
FSA	Food Standards Agency. Established in 2000 as a UK body responsible to the devolved administrations in Scotland, Wales and Northern Ireland as well as the UK Government.
High Level Committee on Research into TSEs	Established in 1997. Chaired by the Cabinet Secretary, with members comprising the CMO, CSA, OST, MAFF, SEAC, BBSRC, MRC and Number Ten. The Committee looks to ensure that: research strategies in relation to human and animal TSEs are in place and implemented as quickly as possible; all relevant sources of expertise are being engaged; any barriers to progress are identified; and to make regular reports to the Prime Minister.
HSE	Health and Safety Executive.

ILGRA	Interdepartmental Liaison Group on Risk Assessment, set up to keep under review developments in the fields of risk assessment, risk management, risk perception and risk communication.
Incubation period	Period between infection and clinical manifestation of disease.
LACOTS	Local Authorities Co-ordinating body on food and trading standards.
MAFF	Ministry of Agriculture, Fisheries and Food.
MBM	Meat and bone meal. Animal-derived protein produced by rendering. Used as a protein source in animal feed.
MCA	Medicines Control Agency, an Executive Agency of DH.
MHS	National Meat Hygiene Service. Part of the FSA. Responsible for meat hygiene inspections since 1 April 1995 and enforces the SRM legislation in licensed slaughterhouses.
Ministerial Science Group	Comprises Ministers from each of the Government departments with significant science, engineering or technology activity. Aims to promote a co-ordinated and coherent approach to policy-making in these areas.
MLC	Meat and Livestock Commission. Established under the Agriculture Act 1967.
Modernising Government	The Government's wide-ranging agenda for modernising the country's Public Services.
MRC	Medical Research Council, a non-departmental public body incorporated by Royal Charter in 1920. Accountable to the OST, it funds research at Universities and at its own research units.

National Zoonoses Group	Chaired by the CMO with members from MAFF, FSA, VMD, DH, PHLS, HSE, VLA, the devolved administrations and LACOTS. Promotes sharing of information and co-ordination of activity on matters connected with zoonoses.
NIBSC	National Institute for Biological Standards and Control.
NPU	Neuropathogenesis Unit. A BBSRC/MRC research unit in Edinburgh working on TSEs.
OST	Office of Science and Technology.
OTMS	Over Thirty Months Scheme. Provides for the purchase of cattle over 30 months old presented for slaughter and for the carcasses to be incinerated or rendered and destroyed.
Pathogen	A bacterium, virus or other micro-organism that can cause disease.
Pathogenesis	The manner of development of a disease.
Permanent Secretary	Head of a Civil Service Department.
PHLS	Public Health Laboratory Service. Responsible for the surveillance and monitoring and contributing to the control of communicable diseases in humans. It does this through a network of laboratories, a central reference laboratory , and a communicable disease surveillance centre.
Pre-clinical	When a disease has not progressed far enough to show clear signs and symptoms.
R&D	Research and Development.
Reagent	A substance or mixture for use in chemical analysis or other reactions.

Rendering	Processing offal and other parts of discarded animal carcasses to make MBM. This is achieved by drying/cooking and separating the solid fraction (protein meals) from the melted liquid fraction (tallow and animal fat).
Research Councils	Non-departmental public bodies that fund research, established under the Science and Technology Act 1965 and by Royal Charter (including BBSRC and MRC). Funded by the Office of Science and Technology.
Ruminant	Animal that chews the cud (partly digested food) regurgitated from its rumen (the first compartment of the stomach of a ruminant), and has a stomach of four compartments.
Ruminant feed ban	Introduced by the BSE Order 1988. In effect it banned the use of MBM (unless derived from non-ruminants) in feed for ruminants (mainly cattle and sheep).
S&T	Science and Technology.
SE	Spongiform Encephalopathy.
SEAC	Spongiform Encephalopathy Advisory Committee. Established in 1990 to advise government on matters related to SEs.
SRM	Specified Risk Material. Specified tissues from cattle, sheep and goats banned for consumption.
Surveillance Group for Diseases and Infections in Animals	Chaired by the CVO, with membership from MAFF, DH, VMD, FSA, PHLS and the devolved administrations. Aims to co-ordinate surveillance activity for zoonoses.
SVS	State Veterinary Service, part of MAFF.
TSE	Transmissible Spongiform Encephalopathy. Disease of the neurological system. Spongy degeneration of the brain with progressive dementia. Examples in humans include CJD and kuru. Among animals: scrapie and BSE.

TSE Research Funders' Group	Members drawn from MAFF, DH, BBSRC, MRC, the devolved administrations, HAS, OST and the Wellcome Trust. Aim is to co-ordinate TSE research activities.
vCJD	Variant CJD. Identified in 1996 as a previously unrecognised form of CJD, having a novel pathology and consistent disease pattern. Exposure to BSE is the most likely explanation for the emergence of the disease.
VIC	Veterinary Investigation Centres. Now part of the VLA in England and Wales. In Scotland they come under the Scottish Agricultural College (part-funded by the Scottish Executive) and are known as Disease Surveillance Centres.
VLA	Veterinary Laboratories Agency. Created in 1995 as a result of the amalgamation of the CVL and 14 VICs. The VLA's purpose is to provide MAFF with specialist veterinary, scientific and technical support, consultancy and surveillance in the fields of animal health and welfare, food safety and the environment. The Agency also delivers services and products to other public and private sector organisations on a commercial basis.
VMD	Veterinary Medicines Directorate, a MAFF agency.
Wellcome Trust	A large charity that funds research.
Whitehall	A collective term for the major Government Departments.
Zoonosis	Animal disease which can be transmitted to humans.

ANNEX VI

STATEMENT BY THE RT. HON NICK BROWN, MINISTER OF AGRICULTURE, FISHERIES AND FOOD AT THE PUBLICATION OF THE BSE INQUIRY REPORT, 26 OCTOBER 2000

<u>Extract from Hansard</u>

The Minister of Agriculture, Fisheries and Food (Mr Nick Brown): With permission, Mr Speaker, I wish to make a statement on the report of the BSE Inquiry, chaired by Lord Phillips of Worth Matravers.

Today, the Government are publishing the report, and I want to announce our initial response and to outline a package of measures for the benefit of people suffering from variant CJD and their families, as well as the families of people who have already died of the disease. This is not however the occasion to announce the Government's substantive response to the Inquiry's report. That will come later.

I should like to express the Government's thanks to Lord Phillips, Mrs June Bridgeman and Professor Malcolm Ferguson-Smith for their thorough Inquiry, which has occupied them for the best part of the past three years.

As the Government recognised when setting up the Inquiry, BSE is a national tragedy. To date, 85 definite or probable cases of variant CJD have been reported in the United Kingdom. Of those 85, 80 people have died. An unknown number of cases are yet to come. It is not possible to give precise forecasts because of the many uncertainties about the disease. I know that the whole House will join me in expressing deepest sympathy to those who have fallen victim to variant CJD, and to their families.

BSE has also had a serious impact on many tens of thousands of people whose livelihoods depend on the rearing of livestock and the processing and manufacturing of meat products.

The Inquiry was set up by my right hon. Friends the Members for Copeland (Dr Cunningham) and for Holborn and St Pancras (Mr Dobson) and the then Secretaries of State for Scotland, for Wales and for Northern Ireland. Its remit was to establish and review the history of the emergence and identification of BSE and new variant CJD and to reach conclusions on the adequacy of the response, taking into account the state of knowledge at that time. The Inquiry Report comprises 16 volumes and some 4,000 pages. Volume 1 sets out the key findings and conclusions.

I shall quote directly from the Report's executive summary. The key conclusions are:

> *"BSE developed into an epidemic as a consequence of an intensive farming practice – the recycling of animal protein in ruminant feed. This practice, unchallenged over decades, proved a recipe for disaster.*
>
> *In the years up to March 1996 most of those responsibilities for responding to the challenge posed by BSE emerge with credit. However, there were a number of shortcomings in the way things were done.*

At the heart of the BSE story lie questions of how to handle hazard – a known hazard to cattle and an unknown hazard to humans. The Government took measures to address both hazards. They were sensible measures, but they were not always timely nor adequately implemented and enforced.

The rigour with which policy measures were implemented for the protection of human health was affected by the belief of many prior to early 1996 that BSE was not a potential threat to human life.

The Government was anxious to act in the best interests of human and animal health. To this end it sought and followed the advice of independent scientific experts – sometimes when decisions could have been reached more swiftly and satisfactorily within government.

In dealing with BSE, it was not MAFF's policy to lean in favour of the agricultural producers to the detriment of the consumer.

At times officials showed a lack of rigour in considering how policy should be turned into practice, to the detriment of the efficacy of the measures taken.

At times bureaucratic processes result in unacceptable delay in giving effect to policy.

The Government introduced measures to guard against the risk that BSE might be a matter of life and death not merely for cattle but also for humans, but the possibility of a risk to humans was not communicated to the public or to those whose job it was to implement and enforce the precautionary measures.

The Government did not lie to the public about BSE. It believe that the risks posed by BSE to humans were remote. The Government was preoccupied with preventing an alarmist over-reaction to BSE because it believed that the risk was remote. It is now clear that this campaign of reassurance was a mistake. When on 20 March 1996 the Government announced that BSE had probably been transmitted to humans, the public felt that they had been betrayed. Confidence in government pronouncement about risk was a further casualty of BSE.

Cases of new variant of CJD (vCJD) were identified by the CJD Surveillance Unit and the conclusion that they were probably linked to BSE was reached as early as was reasonably possible. The link between BSE and vCJD is now clearly established, though the manner of infection is not clear."

Those are direct quotations from Lord Phillips's executive summary.

The Government welcome the report. We will be studying its findings with care and looking closely at the lessons that flow from them. It is right that the House, and the wider public, should have the opportunity to do so. They are important findings and they address some fundamental questions about the adequacy of the response to BSE.

The Report contains many lessons from public administration. We will be focusing our response on areas including the implementation of policy decisions; the process of contingency planning; co-ordination across Departments and other agencies; the assessment, management and communication of risk; the role of scientific advisory committees; and the Government's assessment and use of scientific advice.

Even now, there are some unresolved questions about BSE. We do not know with certainty how the disease entered the cattle herd, or why it has been so predominantly a disease affecting this country. Lord Phillips's conclusion is that the origin of BSE is likely to have been a new prion mutation in cattle, or possibly sheep, in the early 1970s. In the light of that conclusion, my right hon. Friend the Secretary of State for Health and I will be commissioning an independent assessment of current scientific understanding, including emerging findings, of the origins of the BSE epidemic. That study will then be considered by the Spongiform Encephalopathy Advisory Committee, and published.

Although it was beyond the remit of the Inquiry to examine current public protection measures, I know that the House will want to know that the chairman of the Food Standards Agency advises that the report gives rise to no immediate need of new food safety measures. He intends to discuss that aspect of the report at the next public meeting of the agency's on-going review of BSE controls.

Both the Spongiform Encephalopathy Advisory Committee and the Food Standards Agency board propose to review relevant elements of the Report. We will take account of any conclusions or advice that they wish to offer in the Government's response to the Report. The same applies to Select Committees.

The Government will announce their substantive response to the Report in the coming months. Following that announcement, the House will have an early opportunity to debate in Government time both the report and the Government's response. However, there is one element in the report that the Government are singling out for attention now: the care of patients suffering from variant CJD and support for the families caring for them.

The needs of variant CJD victims were frequently insufficient addressed, especially in the early days of the disease. The rapidly degenerative nature of variant CJD requires timely and accurate diagnosis and a swift response form local health and social services departments. Patient care has been variable in the past and not always responsive enough to the rapidly changing needs of patients.

My right hon. Friend the Secretary of State for Health issued new guidelines in August to improve the care of variant CJD victims. The Government now intend to go further.

I can tell the House that, given the special circumstances of those patients, my right Hon. Friend will establish a new national fund for the care of victims of variant CJD. The fund will ensure a speedy response to diagnosis and improvements in the quality of care for patients. This package will be co-ordinated through the national CJD surveillance unit in Edinburgh.

The new national care fund will be used to purchase care and equipment appropriate to the individual needs of variant CJD patients. The fund will be held by the CJD surveillance unit care co-ordinator, supported by a new national network of experts available to support local clinicians and local social services caring for patients wherever they live.

My right hon. Friend the Secretary of State for Health met families of variant CJD victims and representatives of the Human BSE Foundation yesterday to discuss the new package of care. Over the next few weeks, his Department will be working with the families affected to refine the package to ensure that it is effective and properly meets the needs of patients.

This dreadful disease has a devastating effect on victims and their families. The families have campaigned for improved diagnosis and care for those who may yet be affected by this national tragedy. I am sure that the House will want to acknowledge the dignified and constructive way in which they have done so.

In addition to the enhanced care package, we are determined to provide appropriate support for those who are suffering from variant CJD, for those who care for them, and for the families of those who have already died.

The Government therefore intend to put in place financial arrangements to benefit sufferers from variant CJD, and their families, taking account of their particular needs in individual cases.

The Government's preferred option would be to establish a compensation scheme, resulting in a special trust fund, which could amount to millions of pounds. There are a number of possible options. We intend to work closely with the families affected to identify the best way forward. The first discussions with the families and their representatives will take place next week.

The Government want to express their appreciation for the co-operation of all witnesses who have been called before the Inquiry. Although the Inquiry team states that – this is a direct quote -

> *"Any who have come to our Report hoping to find villains or scapegoats, should go away disappointed."*

the Report does make a number of specific criticisms of a number of individuals.

I shall not comment on individual cases. The Report contains an annexe listing those who are criticised. Some of the individuals who are criticised also receive praise from the Inquiry, but there is no corresponding list of individuals who are praised. Elsewhere, the report identifies shortcomings that do not amount to criticisms, and therefore do not feature in the annexe. For both these reasons, it is important that the Report is considered in its entirety.

Whenever serving public servants are subjected to criticism by a public inquiry, the question arises whether any form of disciplinary action should be taken. The report states:

> *"If those criticised were misguided, they were nonetheless acting in accordance with what they conceived to be the proper performance of their duties."*

However, mindful of the importance of the issues covered by the inquiry, an independent person, Sheila Forbes, a Civil Service Commissioner, will lead a review and advise accordingly. The Government want the review to be carried out quickly, across the Departments involved.

The devolved Administrations also received the Report and will respond for their interests.

Hon. Members will also wish to know that I am today sending copies of the Report to the European Commission, the European Parliament and the Governments of each European Union member state. In addition, I have arranged for the Report to be placed on the internet, accessible via the Ministry of Agriculture's website.

On taking office in 1997, this Government put consumers at the heart of decision-making on food safety issues. We have established the independent Food Standards Agency. We have opened up our scientific advisory committees, including the appointment of consumer representatives. We put scientific advice to Government in the public domain, encouraging a culture of openness, trusting the public and stimulating informed public debate. The "deregulation culture" that called for a "bonfire of regulations" has been replaced by a proportionate approach that strives for better regulation, with the protection of the public at its heart. We have put in place working arrangements to encourage the sharing of ideas and information between Government Departments and other agencies.

The Inquiry has made a very thorough assessment of the history of BSE and of the response of the Government of the day. It has added greatly to our understanding of this detailed and complex area. Work is already under way across the whole of government to follow up on the Inquiry's findings. Most importantly today, we are setting in hand improved packages of care and arrangements for financial support for victims of variant CJD and their families. I commend the Inquiry's report to the House.

CONSULTATION

1. The Government's Interim Response to the BSE Inquiry Report is available on the Ministry of Agriculture website at:

    www.maff.gov.uk/animalh/bse/inquiry.html

2. The Report of the BSE Inquiry can also be accessed via the internet at:

    www.bseinquiry.gov.uk.html

3. Comments on the Government's response can be sent by e-mail to the following address:

    bseinquiry@acc.maff.gsi.gov.uk

or they can be sent by post to:

> Mark Filley
> BSE Inquiry Liaison Unit
> Ministry of Agriculture, Fisheries and Food
> 1A Page Street
> London SW1P 4PQ

4. Comments can also be sent to the following contacts in the devolved administrations:

    > For Wales:

    > Gwyn Jones
    > Agriculture Policy Division
    > National Assembly for Wales
    > Cathays Park
    > Cardiff CF10 3NQ
    > gwyn.jones2@wales.gsi.gov.uk

    > For Scotland:

    > Michael Garden
    > BSE Inquiry Liaision Unit
    > Scottish Executive Rural Affairs Dept.
    > Room 358d
    > Pentland House
    > 47 Robb's Loan
    > Edinburgh EH14 1TY
    > michael.garden@scotland.gsi.gov.uk

<u>For Northern Ireland:</u>

Wesley Shannon
Department of Agriculture and Rural Development
Room 714, Dundonald House
Upper Newtownards Road
Belfast BT4 3SB
wesley.shannon@dardni.gov.uk

5. When submitting comments, please provide your full name and address and, where appropriate, details of the organisation you represent. A copy of the Government's final response will be sent to you direct, once published.

6. In line with the Government's policy of openness, it is intended at the end of the consultation period to make copies of responses to this consultation exercise publicly available through the main MAFF Library at Whitehall Place (West Block), London, SW1A 2HH. It will be assumed that your response can be made publicly available in this way unless you indicate clearly that you wish all or part of your response to be excluded from this arrangement. The library will supply copies of the responses received on request to personal callers or telephone enquirers (0645 335577 – local call rates will apply). An administrative charge, to cover photocopying and postage costs, will apply.

7. Comments should be submitted by 11 May 2001.

Printed in the UK by The Stationery Office Limited
On behalf of the Controller of Her Majesty's Stationery Office
Dd 5069786   02/01   019585   TJ003559